Quick Reference to Dental Implant Surgery

Quick Reference to Dental Implant Surgery

Mohamed A. Maksoud

WILEY Blackwell

This edition first published 2017
© 2017 John Wiley & Sons, Inc.

Registered Offices
John Wiley & Sons, Inc., 111 River Street, Hoboken, NJ 07030, USA
John Wiley & Sons Ltd, The Atrium, Southern Gate, Chichester, West Sussex, PO19 8SQ, UK

Editorial Office
111 River Street, Hoboken, NJ 07030, USA

For details of our global editorial offices, customer services, and more information about Wiley products visit us at www.wiley.com.

Wiley also publishes its books in a variety of electronic formats and by print-on-demand. Some content that appears in standard print versions of this book may not be available in other formats.

Library of Congress Cataloging-in-Publication Data

Names: Maksoud, Mohamed A., author.
Title: Quick reference to dental implant surgery / by Mohamed A. Maksoud.
Description: Hoboken, NJ : Wiley, 2017. | Includes bibliographical references and index. |
Identifiers: LCCN 2017018828 (print) | LCCN 2017019356 (ebook) | ISBN 9781119290131 (pdf) |
    ISBN 9781119290162 (epub) | ISBN 9781119290124 (pbk.)
Subjects: | MESH: Dental Implantation–methods | Dental Implants
Classification: LCC RK667.I45 (ebook) | LCC RK667.I45 (print) | NLM WU 640 | DDC 617.6/93–dc23
LC record available at https://lccn.loc.gov/2017018828

Cover image: © alexmit/123RF
Cover design by Wiley

Set in 10/12.5pt WarnockPro by Aptara Inc., New Delhi, India
Printed and bound in Malaysia by Vivar Printing Sdn Bhd

10 9 8 7 6 5 4 3 2 1

To my parents, I know you would be proud of me today. To my wife, thank you for being my best friend.

Contents

About the Author

Mohamed A. Maksoud graduated from Tufts University School of Dental Medicine in Boston, where he earned a Doctor of Dental Medicine degree in addition to a postgraduate periodontology specialty.

He served as faculty member in multiple dental institutions in the United States and abroad, and he is currently at Harvard University School of Dental Medicine in Boston.

Dr. Maksoud is board certified by the American Board of Implant Dentistry, and he is a Diplomate of the International Congress of Oral Implantology.

He has published numerous articles and book chapters in the field of implant dentistry, besides presentations at national and international dental conventions. He is actively involved in teaching training seminars and continuing education courses on dental implants to dentists worldwide, in addition to research and clinical trials in tissue engineering and implant dentistry.

Preface and Introduction

Implantology at present is arguably the most significant discipline in dentistry. It has become a source of intellectual pursuit and patient referrals. Advances in all areas of implant dentistry are occurring at record paces. In the current medico-legal climate, it is important that all practitioners, especially those starting out in implant dentistry, become knowledgeable in all areas. The values of adding skills to one's present capabilities are inestimable. Implantology is one such skill. It offers treatment modalities and techniques of broad and varied interests to all practitioners who wish to work alone or to join others in team efforts.

This book will serve as a unique tool for dental professionals to become proficient in the field of implant dentistry. It illustrates a smooth and systematic approach to all fields in surgical implantology from case selection and diagnostic aids to surgical principles, treatment modalities, and complications. The objective of the book is to provide the reader with a quick and easy navigation guide in a table-based format, with recommendations at the end of each section. It can serve as a teaching reference in dental teaching institutions for dental students and residents, or as a companion in a clinical practice for beginning and advanced implant dentists.

1

Case Selection and Diagnosis

Part A: Medical Consideration in Implant Dentistry

1 Commonly Ordered Blood Tests in Implant Dentistry[1]

Blood test	Normal	Clinical significance
Hematocrit (Hct)	Female: 36–46% Male: 42–52%	Low values: Anemia; monitor for fatigue, dyspnea, tachycardia, and tachypnea.
Hemoglobin (Hgb)	Female: 12–15 g/dl Male: 14–17 g/dl	Low values: Anemia; monitor for fatigue, dyspnea, tachycardia, and tachypnea.
Red blood cell (RBC) count	Female: 4–5.5 million/mm^3 Male: 4.5–6.2 million/mm^3	Low values: Anemia; monitor for fatigue, dyspnea, tachycardia, and tachypnea.
		High values: In chronic obstructive pulmonary disease (COPD), this may indicate polycythemia, a compensation for pulmonary dysfunction that makes blood thicker, increases risk of cerebrovascular accident (CVA).
Total white blood cell (WBC) count	5000–10,000/mm^3	>10,000 indicates systemic infection (more than just local colonization).
Platelets and thrombocytes	200,000–500,000/mm^3	30,000–50,000: Risk of internal hemorrhage.
Erythrocyte sedimentation rate (ESR)	Female: 1–25 mm/h Male: 0–17 mm/h	Bad if elevated. Used to diagnose, or follow the course of, inflammatory diseases (e.g., rheumatic conditions).

(continued)

Quick Reference to Dental Implant Surgery, First Edition. Mohamed A. Maksoud.
© 2017 John Wiley & Sons, Inc. Published 2017 by John Wiley & Sons, Inc.

Blood test	Normal	Clinical significance
Creatinine	Female: 0.6–1.2 mg/dl Male: 0.5–1.1 mg/dl	Renal function measure: High values are bad.
		May indicate nephropathy, or end-stage renal disease.
Potassium (K)	3.5–5.0 mEq/l	Results of low K: Ventricular arrhythmias.
		Results of high K: Ventricular arrhythmias and asystole.
Calcium (Ca)	8.2–10.2 mg/dl	Results of low Ca: Osteoporosis, muscle spasms or tetany, calcium deposits in tissue, cardiac arrhythmia, and asystole.
		Results of high Ca: thirst, polyuria, renal stones, decreased muscle tone, tachycardia, cardiac arrhythmia, and asystole.
Sodium (Na)	136–145 mEq/l	Results of low Na: postural hypotension, abdominal cramps, headache, fatigue, and weakness.
		Results of high Na: edema and tachycardia.
Fasting blood glucose (FBG)	70 to 99 mg/dL	100 to 125 mg/dL: Impaired fasting glucose (pre-diabetes).
		>126 mg/dL: Diabetes.
Serum c-telopeptide collagen	Adult male 18–29 Years 87–1200 pg/mL 30–39 Years 70–780 pg/mL 40–49 Years 60–700 pg/mL 50–68 Years 87–345 pg/mL Adult female 18–29 Years 60–640 pg/mL 30–39 Years 60–650 pg/mL 40–49 Years 40–465 pg/mL	High in osteoporosis, osteopenia, and primary hyperthyroidism.
Alkaline phosphates	30–120 IU/L	High values: liver disease, osteoclastic activity, Paget's disease, bone cancer, and osteoporosis.

Blood test	Normal	Clinical significance
Prothrombin time (PT)	1–18 sec	Measures extrinsic clotting of blood.
		Prolonged in liver disease, impaired vitamin K production, and surgical trauma with blood loss.
Partial thromboplastin time (PTT)	By laboratory control	Measures intrinsic clotting of blood and congenital clotting disorders.
		Prolonged in hemophilia A, B, and C.
International Normalized Ratio (INR)	Without anticoagulant therapy: 1 Anticoagulant therapy target range: 2–3	Measures extrinsic clotting function. Increased with anticoagulant therapy.
Bleeding time (BT)	1–6 min	Measures quality of platelets.
		Prolonged in thrombocytopenia.

A   Recommendations

1. Low platelet count and abnormal clotting tests in addition to abnormal BT, PT, PTT, or INR value is a contraindication in implant surgery, especially in a sinus grafting procedure, due to the possibility of uncontrolled bleeding.

2. Abnormal c-telopeptide values related to the use of oral or systemic bisphosphonates should be considered prior to implant surgery.
3. Consult with a physician in writing regarding any abnormal values, and attach a copy of the blood test results.

2   ASA Classifications

- ASA Physical Status 1: A normal healthy patient.
- ASA Physical Status 2: A patient with mild systemic disease.
- ASA Physical Status 3: A patient with severe systemic disease.
- ASA Physical Status 4: A patient with severe systemic disease that is a constant threat to life.
- ASA Physical Status 5: A moribund patient who is not expected to survive without the operation.
- ASA Physical Status 6: A declared brain-dead patient whose organs are being removed for donor purposes.

A   Recommendations

- ASA Status 1 and 2 can be treated in a dental office.
- ASA Status 3 and 4 should be treated in an in-patient facility.

3   Medical Conditions[1]

A   Scleroderma

1. A multisystem disorder characterized by inflammatory, vascular, and sclerotic changes of the skin and various internal organs, especially the lungs, heart, and gastrointestinal tract.
2. Typical clinical features in the facial region are a masklike appearance, thinning of the lips, microstomia, sclerosis of the sublingual ligament, and indurations of the tongue.
3. The symptoms cause the skin of the face and lips as well as the intraoral mucosa to become taut, thereby hindering dental treatment and complicating or even preventing the insertion of dental prostheses.
4. No controlled studies were found for scleroderma to demonstrate any positive or negative effects on the outcome of implant therapy.

B   Oral Lichen Planus (OLP)

1. A common T-cell-mediated autoimmune disease of unknown cause that affects stratified squamous epithelium exclusively.
2. OLP has been considered a contraindication for the placement of dental implants possibly because of the altered capacity of the oral epithelium to adhere to the titanium surface.
3. OLP as a risk factor for implant surgery and long-term success cannot be properly assessed.

C   Ectodermal Dysplasia (ED)

1. A hereditary disease characterized by congenital dysplasia of one or more ectodermal structures.
2. Common extra- and intraoral manifestations include defective hair follicles and eyebrows, frontal bossing, nasal bridge depression, protuberant lips, hypo- or anodontia, conical teeth, and generalized spacing.
3. Most search results for ED were case reports demonstrating treatment success with dental implants.
4. A few larger case series report survival and success rates of implants in such patients. All studies reported significantly lower survival and success rates in the maxilla than in the mandible.

D   Sjögren's Syndrome (SS)

1. A chronic autoimmune disease affecting the exocrine glands, primarily the salivary and lacrimal glands. The etiology of SS is far from being understood.
2. The most common symptoms of SS are extreme tiredness, along with dry eyes (keratoconjunctivitis sicca) and dry mouth (xerostomia).
3. Xerostomia can eventually lead to difficulty in swallowing, severe and progressive tooth caries, or oral infections.
4. Currently, there is no cure for SS, and treatment is mainly palliative.

5. Literature on implant performance in patients with SS is scarce. There are no controlled studies available, and only one case series study with eight patients included was found. The eight patients in this study were all women receiving a total of 54 implants (18 in the maxilla and 36 in the mandible) with a machined surface. Seven of these implants (12.9%) were found not to be osseointegrated at abutment connection. During the first year of function, two additional implants in the mandible were lost, resulting in an implant-based failure rate of 16.7% (the patient-based rate was 50%; four patients out of eight lost at least one implant).

E Crohn's Disease

1. An idiopathic chronic inflammatory disorder of the gastrointestinal tract that may also involve the oral cavity.
2. The disease process is characterized by recurrent exacerbations and remissions.
3. The literature regarding the performance of dental implants in patients with Crohn's disease is scarce. In a retrospective study with observation up to 1 week after second-stage surgery, two of three patients with Crohn's disease had implant failures (3 out of 10 inserted implants were lost). The authors speculated that the presence of antibody–antigen complexes might lead to autoimmune inflammatory processes in several parts of the body, including the bone–implant interface. However, in both of these patients with early implant failures, other medical and local risk factors were also present: claustrophobia, smoking, and poor bone quantity. In a follow-up study, patients treated from 1982 to 2003 were evaluated to assess the influence of systemic and local factors on the occurrence of early implant failures. Crohn's disease was significantly related to early implant failure. Unfortunately, the authors did not provide the exact number of patients with Crohn's disease treated or the number of implant failures in these patients. In a recent prospective study from the same group, the influence of various systemic and local factors on the occurrence of early failures was once more evaluated. This time, the implants had a modified, oxidized titanium surface. Between November 2003 and June 2005, 11 of 12 implants placed in patients with Crohn's disease integrated successfully.

F Transplantation (Heart, Liver, and Renal Transplant)

1. Patients receiving transplanted organs generally undergo long-term immunosuppressive therapy, usually consisting of cyclosporine combined with steroids, which have anti-inflammatory properties. Several animal studies have demonstrated that cyclosporine may negatively influence bone healing around dental implants and may even impair the mechanical retention of dental implants previously integrated in bone.
2. In human studies, there is no information available in the literature addressing heart or renal transplantations and the performance of subsequently placed or already present dental implants. There is one case report describing the placement of two implants 6 months after liver transplantation, providing anecdotal evidence of stability 10 years after insertion.

G   Diabetes or Insulin Therapy or Glucose Intolerance

1. Type 1 (insulin-dependent) diabetes mellitus is caused by an autoimmune reaction destroying the beta cells of the pancreas, leading to insufficient production of insulin. Type 2 (non-insulin-dependent) diabetes mellitus is viewed as a resistance to insulin in combination with an incapability to produce additional compensatory insulin. Type 2 diabetes is often linked to obesity and is the predominant form, notably in the adult population in need of implant therapy.
2. Diabetes is associated with various systemic complications, including retinopathy, nephropathy, neuropathy, micro- and macrovascular disturbances, and impaired wound healing.
3. In the oral cavity, xerostomia, caries, and periodontitis have been linked to diabetes. The increased susceptibility to periodontitis is thought to be due to a negative influence of diabetes on inflammatory mechanisms and apoptosis, resulting in a deregulated host defense, deficits in wound healing, and microvascular problems.

H   Osteoporosis or Osteoporotic

1. This is a decrease in bone mass and bone density and an increased risk and/or incidence of fracture. However, it has been noted that subjects without fractures also may have lost a significant amount of bone, while many patients with fractures display levels of bone mass similar to those of control subjects. Thus, definitions of osteoporosis based on reduced bone mass or nonviolent fracture are not perfectly synonymous. In addition, the relationship between skeletal and mandibular or maxillary bone mass is limited.
2. The World Health Organization has established diagnostic criteria for osteoporosis based on bone density measurements determined by dual energy X-ray absorptiometry: A diagnosis of osteoporosis is made if the bone mineral density level is 2.5 standard deviations below that in a mean young population.

I   Bisphosphonates

1. Bisphosphonates reduce or even suppress osteoclast function and can therefore be used in the treatment of various disorders causing abnormal bone resorption, including malignancies affecting the bone, such as multiple myeloma and bone metastases of breast and prostate cancer.
2. Patients receiving systemic bisphosphonates combined with steroids are not good candidates for implant treatment due to lack of trabeculation.

4   Recommendations for Medical Consideration in Implant Dentistry

Medical condition	Surgical consideration	Recommendations
Diabetes mellitus	Hypoglycemia due to lack of food intake	• Supplemental antibiotics • Adjust insulin dose • Steroids
Osteoporosis	Possible jaw fracture due to lack of ossification	Assess severity of bone loss through blood Ca level

Medical condition	Surgical consideration	Recommendations
Vitamin D deficiency	Reduced bone trabeculation	Assess severity of bone loss through blood Ca level
Hyperthyroidism and fibrous dysplasia	Affect trabecular pattern Ground glass appearance	• Maximize the number and length of implants • Conservative surgical approach • Longer osseo-integration period • Progressive loading • Bone and sinus augmentation (to ensure graft viability, augment using a higher percentage of autogenous graft than allograft and xenograft)
Paget's disease and multiple myeloma	Cotton wool appearance Increased Serum Alkaline Phosphatase and Blood Calcium Level	No implants
Scleroderma	Microstomia Taut intraoral mucosa	No implants
Oral lichen planus	Autoimmune inflammation of the mucosa	No implants
Sjögren's syndrome	Xerostomia	No implants
Crohn's disease	Autoimmune inflammation of the mucosa	No implants
Liver, kidney, and pancreatic transplant	Cyclosporine taken as an immunosuppressant affects implant-to-bone healing	No implants
Cardiovascular disease	Blood thinners	Monitor and adjust
HIV	Immunocompromised and xerostomia	No implants
Systemic bisphosphonates combined with steroids	Lack of bone trabeculation	No implants

Part B: Radiographic Examination and Imaging Modalities[2-4]

1 Imaging Strategies

Several radiographic examinations are used for preoperative assessment of dental implant sites. Each examination has specific indications, advantages, and disadvantages; however, a perfect imaging examination for dental implant treatment planning does not exist.

A Plain-Film Radiography

1. This term refers to projection images obtained with a stationary x-ray source and area detector.
2. Plain-film images represent the entire volume through which the x-ray beam is transmitted and is subject to differential magnification, geometrical distortion, and anatomic superimposition.

Intraoral radiography

1. Periapical intraoral radiography provides images of limited dentoalveolar regions that have excellent contrast resolution with minimal distortions.
2. Images are taken using film-holding devices to allow regional visualizations of vertical and anteroposterior bounds of residual alveolar ridges and identifications of adjacent anatomical structures.
3. The technique is the most widely available, inexpensive, and common initial dental radiographic examination for implant site assessment. The technique, however, is highly operator dependent and requires a moderate level of patient compliance to provide images with minimal geometrical distortions.
4. The greatest limitation of this strategy is the lack of cross-sectional information to access bone volume.
5. Occlusal radiography provides information on the general shape of the residual dental arch and maximum buccolingual dimension of the alveolar ridge; also, occlusal radiography has been proposed as a supplement to periapical radiography for implant assessments. Occlusal radiography, however, provides no information in addition to that provided by dental study models, and its use is not, therefore, justified for implant site assessments.

Cephalometric radiography

1. Cephalometrics includes two-dimensional lateral representations of the anteroposterior and vertical relationships of the maxillary and mandibular dental arches. Edentulous spaces in the midline are represented as cross-sectional images that can be calibrated to provide accurate measurement of buccolingual as well as vertical bone dimensions of the anterior residual alveolar ridge. Equipment for cephalometric radiography is readily available, and cephalometric images are relatively easy to obtain and of low cost.

2. The use of these images is limited, however, in that they provide uniformly magnified images of midline structures only. Although oblique, lateral cephalograms are used to image anterolateral segments, the alveolar process is often obscured by the superimposition of teeth adjacent to the edentulous alveolus.

B Rotational Panoramic Radiography

1. Panoramic radiographs provide information on the inferior alveolar canals and maxillary sinuses, and they may show pathologic conditions not demonstrated on complete, intraoral radiographic examinations.
2. Panoramic radiography is commonly available, is relatively low cost, provides information on both dental arches, and is useful in the initial diagnostic phase of implant planning.
3. By calculating the ratio between image dimensions and known dimensions of radiopaque markers on a radiographic stent, estimates of the available vertical distances between the alveolar crest and anatomic structures can be estimated at specific positions in a panoramic image.
4. Many factors, however, limit the accuracy and reliability of this calculation. These include patient-positioning errors, inherent distortions related to equipment differences, discrepancies between the shape of the dental arch and focal trough, and beam angulation.
5. A major limitation of panoramic radiography is that buccolingual assessments cannot be made. Because of its inherent limitations, panoramic radiography is considered unsuitable as a single imaging source for dental implant site assessment.

C Cross-sectional Imaging Techniques

1. Cross-sectional imaging techniques produce in-focus, thin-section images. Cross-sectional images can be produced with conventional tomography, panoramic-based scanography and tomography, cone beam computed tomography (CBCT), and computed tomography (CT).
2. CT scanners are most commonly used in medical radiology departments and hospitals.
3. Tomographic images can also be obtained with magnetic resonance (MR) imaging.
4. Tomographic techniques produce multiple, contiguous image sections (slices), with minimal distortions and uniform thicknesses and magnifications. In addition, images can be reconstructed such that they are perpendicular to each other.
5. The main advantage of tomographic images for implant dentistry is that they minimize or eliminate anatomic superimposition.

Conventional tomography

1. In conventional tomography, the x-ray source and the receptor move in synchrony and in opposite directions to each other about a fixed fulcrum, and this results in the blurring of structures outside the image plane, which is at the level

of the fulcrum. For implant dentistry, this provides uniformly magnified images in two dimensions, usually sagittal and coronal (cross-sectional). A limitation of this technique is that it produces images of limited regions (a few teeth) of a single dental arch.

2. Only objects within the specific region of interest are in focus. Usually, stents with radiopaque markers are needed to confirm the positions of imaged sites.

3. Because of blurring outside the region in focus, it is often difficult to identify structures and interpret the images.

Panoramic-based tomography

1. Some panoramic units use x-ray beam motions and area receptors to produce planar or curved (scanogram) tomographic images. Units vary markedly in the anatomic localization methods used, the number and thickness of tomographic slices, and the resultant image magnifications.

2. Images are often extremely wide compared with the area under study, may not cover the region of interest sufficiently, and suffer from blur, making interpretation of images difficult. Although this technique can be helpful in preliminary evaluations of specific implant sites, the technique is time-consuming, and multiple inter- or intra-arch implant site assessments require multiple exposures.

Computed tomography

1. Mostly uses fan-beam radiation and multiple detector arrays. Usually, one source of fan-beam radiation is used. The user makes selections to define the spatial resolution, field of view (FOV), and image sharpness. From the volume of data that is collected, mathematical formulas are used to reconstruct volumetric and/or multiplanar images. The multiplanar reconstructions can have various image thicknesses (several millimeters to tenths of millimeters) and be in any image plane (sagittal, coronal, axial, or any plane in between). Images are undistorted, are calibrated for dimensional accuracy, and have high soft tissue and hard tissue contrast resolution.

2. CT is relatively expensive, and it is usually available in hospitals and medical imaging centers only.

Cone beam computed tomography

1. CBCT differs from CT in that it uses a single x-ray source that produces a cone beam of radiation (rather than a fan beam, as with CT). CBCT uses a single, relatively inexpensive, flat-panel or image-intensifier radiation detector.

2. CBCT imaging is performed using a rotating platform to which the x-ray source and detector are fixed. The x-ray source and detector rotate around the object being scanned, and multiple, sequential, planar projection images are acquired in an arc of 180° or greater and are mathematically reconstructed into a volumetric dataset.

3. Many CBCT devices are now multimodal, providing panoramic and cephalometric imaging. Most have a low footprint suitable for dental office placement,

are technically as easy to operate as panoramic units, allow collimation of the beam to the region of interest to reduce patient radiation exposures, and produce submillimeter-resolution images of high quality. Although CBCT images have high spatial resolution, the data from which images are created contains considerable noise caused by scattered radiation.

4. Both CT and CBCT volumetric datasets can be exported in DICOM (Digital Imaging and Communications in Medicine) format and imported into third-party software that is specifically designed for implant treatment planning. With such software, various three-dimensional and cross-sectional images can be created. It is also possible to create virtual image-displays and simulated implant placement, and to use the software for computer-guided surgery.

5. In comparison with conventional dental imaging, volumetric datasets provide additional information that can be used for more sophisticated analyses and expanded, treatment-planning options that result in higher likelihoods for achieving satisfactory prosthetic results.

6. For use in implant dentistry, a major advantage of CBCT compared with CT is that CBCT equipment is usually far less expensive than CT equipment. Another advantage is that CBCT software for use in planning implants is usually much easier to use and far more useful than is software available with CT. The primary disadvantages of both CT and CBCT are their relatively higher effective radiation exposures and additional costs compared with plain, panoramic, and some other cross-sectional radiographic methods.

Advantages of CBCT	Disadvantages of CBCT
Multiplanar reconstruction.	Limited soft tissue visualization.
Significantly less radiation compared with other 3D advanced imaging modalities (e.g., medical CT).	Some CBCT machines produce an increased radiation exposure compared with selected intraoral and panoramic radiographs.
Fast, efficient, in-office modality.	
Interactive treatment planning.	Limited bone density measurements.
Adequate for bone-grafting assessment.	Artifacts created by metal subjects (e.g., porcelain fused-to-metal [PFM] crowns, dental implants).
Computer-aided surgery.	
	Third-party software applications and 3D models are additional expenses.
	Liability and extra cost.

MR imaging

1. With MR imaging (which does not use ionizing radiation), cross-sectional images (suitable for dental implant treatment planning) can be created.

2. The limitations of these images for dental implant imaging are the increased imaging scan times, dentists' unfamiliarity with MR images, and higher costs.

2   Radiographic Examination and Imaging Modalities

Modality	Mode of action	Magnifications and distortion	Radiation	In-office or out-of-office facility	Advantages and disadvantages in implant dentistry
Periapical	X-ray head	None Single tooth area	Light	In office	Only in single implant cases
Panoramic	Panorex	Distorted image Overlap of syloid process of the mandible on maxillary sinuses Overlap of the cervical vertebrae on the anterior teeth	Moderate	In office	For diagnostic purposes only
Occlusal	X-ray head	None Limited to occlusal plane view	Light	In office	No benefits
CT	Multiple x-ray heads produce fan-beam projections Slices staked to form 3D image	None	High	Out of office	High-radiation dose with scattered radiation High cost and patient inconvenience
CBCT	Single x-ray head produces cone beam projections 3D image sliced	None	Low	In office	Low cost Convenient Less radiation exposure
MR imaging	Magnetic resonance imaging	None	None	Out of office	No benefits
Cephalometric	X-ray head	Yes	High	In office	No benefits

A   Terms Used in Digital Radiography

Pixel	The smallest controllable element of a picture represented on the screen in a two-dimensional grid.
Voxel	The smallest controllable element of a picture represented on the screen in a three-dimensional grid.
DICOM	Digital Imaging and Communication in Medicine.
FOV	Field of view.
6-inch FOV	Produces an image of teeth sextants or an arch.
9-inch FOV	Produces an image of dentition and orbit.
12-inch FOV	Produces an image of the whole skull.

B   Indications of CBCT in the Maxillofacial Region

* Evaluation of the jaw bones to assess the feasibility of placing dental implants at specific sites in the jaws. This ensures that every possible precaution has been made to reduce the risk of involvement of the nerves in the lower jaw, and the sinuses and nose in the upper jaw.
* Evaluation of the status of previously placed implants.
* Evaluation of the hard tissue (bones) of the temporomandibular joint (TMJ).
* Evaluation of abnormalities (pathology) in or affecting the bones.
* Evaluation of the extent of alveolar ridge resorption.
* Assessment of relevant structures prior to orthodontic treatment, such as the presence and position of impacted canine and third molar teeth.
* Assessing symmetry of the face (cephalometrics).
* Assessing the airway space (sleep apnea).
* To permit 3D reconstructions of the bones or the fabrication of a biomodel of the face and jaws.
* Assessing the mandibular nerve prior to the removal of impacted teeth, especially the lower wisdom teeth.

C   CBCT versus Dental X-Ray

CBCT	**Dental X-Rays**
Cone beam CT images provide undistorted, or accurate, dimensional views of the jaws.	Panoramic images, by contrast, are both magnified and distorted.
Distortion is the unequal magnification of different parts of the same image.	Magnification by itself is not a problem, as long as one knows or can calculate the magnification factor.

In addition, CT images can provide cross-sectional (buccolingual), axial, coronal, sagittal, and panoramic views.

With CT, it is possible to separate the various structures, for example the left condyle from the right one.

Due to distortion, panoramic images are notoriously unreliable to use for making measurements.

A panoramic film provides an image of only one dimension, namely a mesio-distal or antero-posterior perspective. In a panoramic image, all the structures between the x-ray tube and the image detector are superimposed on one another.

D   CBCT Compared to Tomography

CBCT

CBCT can be performed within a 10–40 sec range, depending on the region being imaged and on the desired quality of the image. CBCT also provides stronger indication of bone quality.

The equipment is substantially lighter and smaller.

Cone beam CTs have better spatial resolution (i.e., smaller pixels).

No special electrical requirements are needed.

No floor strengthening is required.

The room does not need to be cooled.

Very easy to operate and maintain; little technician training is required.

Some cone beam manufacturers and vendors are dedicated to the dental market. This makes for a greater appreciation of the dentist's needs.

In the majority of cone beam CTs, the patient is seated, as compared with lying down in a medical CT unit.

Tomography

Tomography, on the other hand, provides direct (as opposed to reconstructed) cross-sectional, sagittal, and coronal views. The disadvantage of plain-film tomography is that it requires much more chair time than CT. Thus, it can be especially difficult to perform on patients who are unable to sit or hold still for a period of time.

Cost of equipment is approximately 3–5 times less than that of traditional medical CT.

Plain-film tomography has lower contrast resolution, which means less discrimination between different tissue types (i.e., bone, teeth, and soft tissue).

CBCT virtually eliminates claustrophobia and greatly enhances patient comfort and acceptance.

The upright position is also thought by many to provide a more realistic picture of condylar positions during a TMJ examination.

The lower cost of the machine may be passed on to the patient in the form of lower fees.

Both jaws can be imaged at the same time (depending on the specific cone beam machine).

Radiation dose is considerably less than with a medical CT.

3 Principles of Imaging for Dental Implant Assessment, with Recommendations

1. Images should have appropriate diagnostic quality and not contain artifacts that compromise anatomic-structure assessments.
2. Images should extend beyond the immediate area of interest to include areas that could be affected by implant placements.
3. Practitioners should have appropriate training in operating radiographic equipment and competence in interpreting images from the modality used. This training and competence should be maintained through continuing dental education courses. Such training should include a thorough review of normal maxillofacial anatomy, common anatomic variants, and imaging signs of diseases and abnormalities. This is particularly important for CT and CBCT imaging because of the complexity of structures within the expanded FOVs.
4. The goal of radiographic selection criteria is to identify appropriate imaging modalities that complement the goals at each stage of implant therapy. The use of specific imaging is based on professional judgment. Professional judgment varies depending on the skill, competence, knowledge, and experience of the clinician.
5. Specific considerations must include clinical and anatomic complexity, potential risks of complications, and esthetic outcomes.

A Initial Examination

The purposes of the initial radiographic examination are to assess the overall status of the remaining dentition, to identify and characterize the location and nature of the edentulous regions, and to detect regional anatomic abnormalities and pathologies.

Recommendation 1.	Recommendation 2.	Recommendation 3.
Panoramic radiography should be used as the imaging modality of choice in the initial evaluation of the dental implant patient.	Use intraoral periapical radiography to supplement the preliminary information from panoramic radiography.	Do not use cross-sectional imaging, including CBCT, in an initial diagnostic imaging examination.

B Preoperatively

1. Establish the morphologic characteristics of the residual alveolar ridge (RAR). The morphology of the RAR includes considerations of bone volume and quality. Vertical bone height, horizontal width, and edentulous saddle length determine the amount of bone volume available for implant fixture placement. This information is necessary to match the available bone dimensions with the number and physical dimensions of the implant(s). Moderate deficiencies in horizontal and vertical bone may be corrected by augmentation procedures at the time of the osteotomies and fixture placements, whereas severe deficiencies require prior surgical procedures, such as ridge augmentations.

2. Similarly, excessive or irregular vertical alveolar bone may require pre-prosthetic or simultaneous alveoloplasty.

3. Bone quality is considered good when there is enough cortical and trabecular (cancellous) bone to hold the implant securely (which is required for osseointegration), and it is considered poor when there is inadequate oral bone to hold the implant securely. The most commonly used classification system for assessing oral-bone quality for implant placement was introduced in 1985 and uses four radiographic oral-bone classes that are based on visual assessments of the amounts of cortical and trabecular bone. Better assessments of bone quality may influence surgical technique, implant selection (i.e., length, diameter, and type), and the loading protocol.

4. Determine the orientation of the RAR. The orientation and residual topography of the alveolar–basal bone complex must be assessed to determine whether there are variations that could compromise the alignment of the implant fixture with the planned prosthetic restoration. This is particularly important in the mandible (e.g., submandibular gland fossa) and anterior maxilla (e.g., labial cortical bone concavity).

5. Identify local anatomic or pathologic conditions restricting implant placement. In the maxilla, these include the incisor region (nasopalatine fossa and canal, and nasal fossa), canine region (canine fossa and nasal fossa), and premolar/molar region (floor of the maxillary sinus). In the mandible, these include the incisor region (lingual foramen), canine/premolar region (mental foramen), and molar region (submandibular gland fossa, and inferior alveolar [mandibular] canal containing the neurovascular bundle).

6. Match imaging findings to the prosthetic plan. Successful implant treatment planning involves both surgical and prosthetic considerations. Radiographic images are not only used for prosthetic planning but also used to construct templates to guide surgical procedures and implant placements. The use of guided surgery for implant placement is increasing because of a number of clinical advantages, including increased practitioner confidence and reduced operating time. Guided surgery requires imaging capable of providing DICOM data (either CT or CBCT). These data are imported into software programs where interactive surgical and prosthetic tools can provide complex implant "simulations" within a virtual patient.

Recommendation 4.

The radiographic examination of any potential implant site should include cross-sectional imaging orthogonal to the site of interest.

Conventional tomography provides cross-sectional information, but it is technique sensitive and the images are more difficult to interpret than CBCT images. CBCT usually results in lower patient exposures to ionizing radiation than does CT.

Recommendation 5.

CBCT should be considered as the imaging modality of choice for preoperative cross-sectional imaging of potential implant sites.

As with any type of imaging, a patient should be exposed to the least amount of ionizing radiation that is needed to produce CBCT images of acceptable diagnostic quality. This is achieved by careful selection of exposure parameters and FOV. Although the FOV should be limited to the area of interest, the FOV may extend beyond the implant site to include the maxillary sinus or opposing dental arch. CT may be considered when CBCT is unavailable; however, dose-sparing protocols must be used.

The use of CBCT before bone grafting helps define both the donor and recipient sites, allows for improved planning for surgical procedures, and reduces patient morbidities. CBCT is best for the evaluation of volumetric and topographic changes of the restored residual alveolar ridge.

Recommendation 6.
CBCT should be considered when clinical conditions indicate a need for augmentation procedures or site development before placement of dental implants: (1) sinus augmentation, (2) block or particulate bone grafting, (3) ramus or symphysis grafting, (4) assessment of impacted teeth in the field of interest, and (5) evaluation of prior traumatic injury.

Recommendation 7.
CBCT imaging should be considered if bone reconstruction and augmentation procedures (e.g., ridge preservation or bone grafting) have been performed to treat bone volume deficiencies before implant placement.

C Postoperative Imaging

1. The purpose of postoperative imaging after dental implant placement is to confirm the location of the fixture at implant insertion.
2. Later in maintaining implant treatment, imaging is used to assess the bone–implant interface and marginal peri-implant bone height.

Recommendation 8.
In the absence of clinical signs or symptoms, use intraoral periapical radiography for the postoperative assessment of implants. Panoramic radiographs may be indicated for more extensive implant therapy cases.

Recommendation 9.
Use cross-sectional imaging (particularly CBCT) immediately postoperatively only if the patient presents with implant mobility or altered sensation, especially if the fixture is in the posterior mandible.

Recommendation 10.
Do not use CBCT imaging for periodic review of clinically asymptomatic implants. Finally, implant failure, owing to either biological or mechanical causes, requires a complete assessment to characterize the existing defect; plan for surgical removal and corrective procedures, such as ridge preservation or bone augmentation; and identify the effect of surgery or the defect on adjacent structures.

Recommendation 11.
Cross-sectional imaging, optimally CBCT, should be considered if implant retrieval is anticipated.

Recommendation 12.

The decision to order a CBCT scan must be based on the patient's history and clinical examination, and justified on an individualized needs basis that demonstrates that the benefits to the patient outweigh the potential risks of the patient's exposure to ionizing radiation, especially in the case of children or young adults and large FOV scans. Because the 3D information obtained with CBCT cannot be obtained with other 2D imaging modalities, it is virtually impossible to predict which treatment cases would not benefit from having this additional information before obtaining it.

Based on the available evidence and the type of information acquired with 3D imaging modalities, the consensus panel suggests that the use of CBCT should be considered as an imaging alternative before cases where the proposed implant receptor or bone augmentation site(s) are suspect, and conventional radiography may not be able to assess the true regional 3D anatomical presentation as indicated here:

- Computer-aided implant planning and placement, including flapless techniques (e.g., interactive treatment planning software applications, surgical guides, and navigation systems).
- Implant placement in a highly esthetic zone or where concavities, ridge inclination, inadequate bone volume or quality, undeterminable proximity to vital structures, and/or insufficient inter-radicular spacing are suspected.

Recommendations 13.

The use of CBCT requires a specific skill set that until recently has not been taught in dental schools at either the undergraduate or postgraduate levels. Therefore, it is also recommended that clinicians who are providing dental implant procedures for their patients become knowledgeable in 3D diagnosis and treatment planning concepts, and become familiar with interactive treatment planning software applications.

Protocols. 3D imaging technology does not supersede sound surgical and restorative/prosthetic fundamentals.

Clinicians should understand that the scan process often starts before the scan itself. Diagnostic wax-ups, mounted articulated study casts, and the use of scanning templates help to improve the diagnostic accuracy of the CBCT data as it relates to the desired implant placement or ancillary grafting procedure. The use of scanning and surgical templates helps to improve surgical accuracy, reduce postoperative morbidity, and aid in the restorative phase of treatment.

- Pre- and postadvanced bone grafting evaluation (e.g., sinus lift, ridge splitting, and block grafting).
- History or suspected trauma to the jaws, foreign bodies, maxillofacial lesions, and/or developmental defects.
- Evaluation of postimplant complications (e.g., postoperative neurosensory impairment, osteomyelitis, and acute rhinosinusitis).

It is important to keep in mind that the smallest possible FOV should be used and the entire image volume should be interpreted.

Part C: Surgical Stents[5–7]

1 Surgical Stent Types

A Type 1: Teeth Occlusal Access Hole

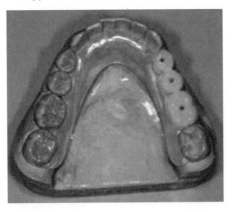

Figure 1.1 Surgical stent with teeth and occlusal access hole.

In Figure 1.1, teeth are set in an ideal diagnostic arrangement, and a hole is drilled through the tooth giving the most ideal placement and angulation for the implant. It allows the surgeon to place the pilot drill through this hole to the tissue and drill a small pilot hole into the bone at this exact location. When the tissue flap is made, the pilot holes are visible and the implant can be placed in this area. A few of the drawbacks are: once the flap is made the stent is no longer useful, and the long axis of the implant is not visually apparent. The buccal flange can be removed, which would aid the surgeon visually if bone grafting or the use of particle bone in areas is needed. It also can be worn by the patient during healing as long as relief is made to the underside so there is no pressure to the ridge during the healing process. The position of the hole in the template determines whether the implant crown will be screw retained or cemented.

B   Type 2: Clear Occlusal Access, No Teeth

Figure 1.2   Surgical stent with clear occlusal access and no teeth.

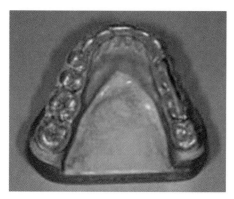

In Figure 1.2, this type of stent defines the outer perimeter of the teeth that have been set in an ideal diagnostic arrangement. It allows the surgeon to flap the tissue and place the stent over the visible bone. The gingival tissue position is also apparent from the facial, giving the surgeon information regarding whether grafted or particle bone is needed in any particular area for proper tissue support or the regeneration of the inner dental papilla. The stent also can be utilized as an impression tray during first-stage surgery in preparation of a temporary prosthesis for placement at second-stage surgery.

C   Type 3: Teeth Barium Coated

Figure 1.3   Surgical stent with teeth and barium coated.

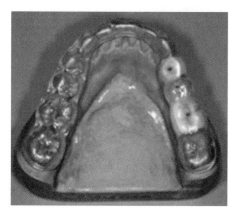

The type of stent in Figure 1.3 is prepared as the "Confined," with the addition of barium placed within the inner. This stent is specifically designed for diagnostics with CBCT.

D Type 4: Clear with Sleeves

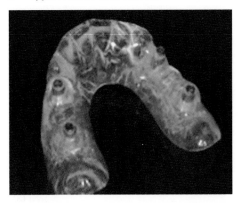

Figure 1.4 Surgical stent clear with sleeves.

The type of stent in Figure 1.4 is prepared as the "Confined" design with metal pins placed into the pilot holes. The facial side of the stent is removed, leaving a lingual wall. This allows the surgeon to flap the tissue and place the stent over the visible bone. The surgeon has open access to the labial side with the aid of these guide pins to maintain a visual parallel path during first-stage surgery. The stent can be used for single-tooth to full-arch implant placement. The stent also can be used as an aid when taking a full panorex. The guide pins will be a visible reference in the early planning stages. The gingival tissue position is apparent from the facial, giving the surgeon information regarding whether grafted or particle bone is needed in any particular area for proper tissue support or the regeneration of the inner dental papilla. The stent also could be utilized as an impression tray during first-stage surgery in preparation of a temporary prosthesis for placement at second-stage surgery.

E Type 5: Clear, No Lingual

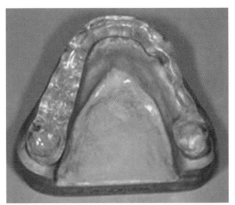

Figure 1.5 Surgical stent clear with no lingual flange.

In Figure 1.5, this type of stent is prepared as the "Parallel Pin" without the addition of the pins, and the lingual is hollowed out.

F   Type 6: Clear, Fully Edentulous

Figure 1.6 Surgical stent clear fully edentulous.

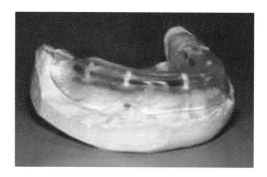

The type of stent in Figure 1.6 is used when a bar or individual abutments will be used for an implant-supported overdenture.

G   Type 7: Opposite-Arch Pins

Figure 1.7 Surgical stent on the opposite arch with pins.

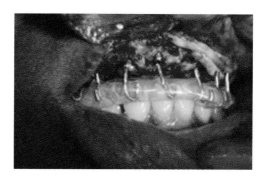

In Figure 1.7, this type of stent is used when no interferences from the stent are desired in the affected surgical site. The stent that is fabricated on the opposite arch has pins that correspond to the implant's location on the opposite (surgical) site.

2 **Comparison of Surgical Stents**

Stent	Access hole diameter	Visibility	Ability to change alignment during drilling	Ability to determine need for bone grafting	Can be used for diagnosis with radiographs and scans	Can be used for impression taking	Can be used as temporary appliance during healing
Type 1: Teeth occlusal access hole	Pilot drill only	Limited	No	Yes	Yes	No	Yes
Type 2: Clear occlusal access, no teeth	Any drill diameter	Unlimited	Yes	Yes	No	Yes	No
Type 3: Teeth barium coated	Any drill diameter	Limited	No	Yes	Yes	No	Yes
Type 4: Clear with sleeves	Pilot drill	Limited	No	Yes	Yes	No	No
Type 5: Clear, no lingual	Any drill diameter	Unlimited	Yes	No	No	No	No
Type 6: Clear, fully edentulous	Pilot drill	Limited	No	No	No	No	No
Type 7: Opposite-arch wires	Any drill diameter	Unlimited	Yes	Yes	No	No	No

3 Recommendations

1. Surgical stents with access holes should be wide enough to accommodate the drills.
2. Patients wearing stents during a CT scan or cone beam tomography taken outside the dental office should be trained first on how to wear the stents. Identify the upper and lower stents to patients.

References

1 Misch CE. Contemporary Implant Dentistry, 3rd ed. Mosby Elsevier, 2008.
2 Tyndall DA, Price JB, Tetradis S Ganz S. Position statement of the American Academy of Oral and Maxillofacial Radiology on selection criteria for the use of radiology in dental implantology with emphasis on cone beam computed tomography. Oral Surg Oral Med Oral Pathol Oral Radiol 2012 Jun;113(6): 817–826.
3 Harris D, Horner K, Gröndahl K, et al. EAO guidelines for the use of diagnostic imaging in implant dentistry 2011: a consensus workshop organized by the European Association for Osseointegration at the Medical University of Warsaw. Clin Oral Implants Res 2012;23:1243–1253.
4 Harris D, Buser D, Dula K, et al. EAO guidelines for the use of diagnostic imaging in implant dentistry. Clin Oral Implants Res 2002;13:566–570.
5 Monson ML. Diagnostic and surgical guides for placement of dental implants. J Oral Maxillofac Surg 52:642–645.
6 Becker CM, Kaiser DA. Surgical guide for dental implant placement. J Prosthet Dent 2000;83:248–251.
7 Almog DM, Torrado E. Fabrication of imaging and surgical guides for dental implants. J Prosthet Dent 2001;85:504–508.

2

Surgical Principles and Protocols

Part A: Scrubbing and Gowning[1]

1 Preparation Prior to Surgical Scrub

- Make sure that your skin and nails are clean. Nails should be short and have no cuticles.
- Inspect hands for cuts and abrasions. Skin should not have open lesions or cracked skin.
- Be sure that your hair is covered by headgear.
- Adjust the water to the comfortable temperature.
- Fingernails should not reach beyond the fingertip to avoid glove puncture.
- Remove all jewelry.
- Adjust your disposable mask. Make sure that the mask is perfectly fitted and you are comfortable with it.

2 Surgical Scrubbing Methods

A Time Method

This surgical scrub method has two subtypes: *complete scrub* and *short scrub*.

- *Complete scrub* takes about five to seven minutes. This is done before the first gowning and gloving, if the gloves have been removed before the gown, if the gloves have a lot of holes between them, if the hands have been contaminated in any other way, and before any emergency surgery procedure.
- *Short scrub* takes about three minutes. This is done to remove bacteria that have emerged from the pores and multiplied while the gloves are on.

B Brush Stroke Method

A number of brush strokes is done for each surface of the fingers, hands, and arms.

Quick Reference to Dental Implant Surgery, First Edition. Mohamed A. Maksoud.
© 2017 John Wiley & Sons, Inc. Published 2017 by John Wiley & Sons, Inc.

3 Steps for Surgical Scrubbing

1. Turn on water, and get the antiseptic solution.
2. Wash hands prior to scrubbing.
3. Clean fingers under running water.
4. Scrub the hands as well as the fingertips.
5. Scrub the left arm and the left elbow.
6. Rinse the brush that is used, and transfer to the other hand.
7. Scrub your right arm and the right elbow area.
8. Rinse.
9. Complete scrub by anatomical timed or stroke count.
10. Scrub the nails of one hand with 30 strokes, all sides of each finger with 20 strokes, the back of the hand with 20 strokes, the palm of the hand with 20 strokes, and the arms with 20 strokes. All strokes should be applied lengthwise.
11. Rinse well.
12. Turn off the water faucet with a brush if the water faucet is hand controlled.
13. Walk to the operating room (OR) with the hands on the level of the heart. Make sure that your scrubbed hands will not touch anything, or it will be considered unsterile and you will need to do the surgical scrubbing again.

4 Drying the Hands

❖ Now you are entering the OR from the scrub area to the sterile back table.
❖ Slightly bend forward, pick up the hand towel from the top of the gown pack, and step back from the table.
❖ Grasp the towel, and open it so that it is folded to double thickness lengthwise.
❖ Do not allow the towel to touch any unsterile object; keep your arms away from your body.
❖ Holding one end of the towel with one of your hands, dry your other hand and arm with a blotting, rotating motion.
❖ Work from your fingertips to the elbow.
❖ Do not retrace any area.
❖ Dry all sides of the fingers, the forearm, and the arms thoroughly.
❖ Grasp the other end of the towel, and dry your other hand and arm in the same manner as above.

5 Gowning

❖ Surgical gowns are folded with the inside facing the scrub person.
❖ This facilitates picking up and donning the gown without touching the outside surface.
❖ If you touch the outside surface of the gown while donning it, the gown is contaminated.
❖ Remember: your hands are not sterile; they are just clean.

* Your scrubbed hands and arms are contaminated if you allow them to fall below waist level or to touch your body.
* With one hand, pick up the entire folded gown from the wrapper by grasping through all layers, being careful to touch only the inside top layer, which is exposed.
* Unfold the gown. Hold the gown away from you, at chest level, to facilitate safe handling without a break in asepsis.
* Grasp the inside shoulder seams, and open the gown with the armholes facing you.
* Slide your arms partway into the sleeves of the gown, keeping your hands at shoulder level away from the body.
* Hold your hands high so the gown does not touch the floor.
* With the assistance of your circulator, slide your arms further into the gown sleeves.

* When the fingertips are even with the proximal edge of the cuff, grasp the inside seam at the juncture of the gown sleeve and cuff, using your thumb and index finger.
* Be careful that no part of your hand protrudes from the sleeve cuff.
* The circulator must continue to assist at this point. He or she positions the gown over your shoulders by grasping the inside surface of the gown at the shoulder seams.
* The circulator then prepares to secure the gown; the neck and back may be secured with a Velcro tab or ties.
* The circulator ties the gown at waist level at the back. This technique prevents the contaminated surfaces at the back of the gown from coming into contact with the front of the gown.

A Gowning: Open Cuff

* The procedure is the same as in the "Gowning" section, except you do *not* grasp the inside seam of the sleeve but allow your hands to protrude from the cuffs of the gown.
* Both you and the circulator must be careful that the gown cuffs are not pulled too high on the wrists.
* The edge of the cuff should be at the distal end of the wrist.

B Final Tie of Gown

* Gloves are on, and you are ready to complete the gown tie with the assistance of the circulator.
* Hold the paper tab: do not pull.
* Gently undo the knot so that you have the other belt in your other hand.
* Hand over the paper tab to the circulator while holding the belt.
* Spin, and the circulator will pull the paper tab.
* Now you tie the knot.

6   De-gowning

With gloves on: untie the waist strap, then remove gloves, then remove gown.

7   Recommendations

a. The above protocol is for an OR setting in the hospital or an outpatient facility.	b. In a dental office, following the above steps is recommended for multiple or invasive implant surgery.

Part B: Surgical Report

The surgical report serves as a comprehensive narrative of the procedure performed by the surgeon in a descriptive and precise manner. As an integral part of the patient file, it serves as a legal document and as a reference for review of any medical practitioner who is involved in the patient's care. In the event of any future complications, the report review can determine the best course of the complication treatment. In dentistry where dental implantologists are involved in invasive procedures of implant and bone surgery, a surgical report is a crucial element of the dental implants practice.

1   Principles

- Date of procedure
- Patient name
- Surgeon
- Assistants
- Preoperative diagnosis
- Postoperative diagnosis
- Procedure
- Procedure in detail
- Premedication
- Time of arrival
- Anesthesia
- Incision
- Flap
- Surgical stent
- Implant
- X-ray films
- Sutures
- Postoperative instructions
- Medications
- Patient condition at dismissal

2   Recommendations

1. A detailed surgical report is a great reference tool for all clinicians involved in implant treatment.

2. In addition, it serves as a legal document in cases involving litigation.

3. See the "Sample Surgical Report" in chapter 6.

Part C: Commonly Used Medications in Implant Dentistry

1 Pain Management

A Mild Pain Management

Drug name	Ingredients	Doses	Directions
Motrin	Ibuprofen	800 mg	One tablet three times a day
Ultracet	Tramadol and acetaminophen	Tramadol 37.5 mg and acetaminophen 325 mg	Two tabs every 4–6 h, not to exceed 8 tabs a day
Tylenol #3	Acetaminophen and codeine	Acetaminophen 300 mg, caffeine 15 mg, and codeine phosphate 30 mg	One tab every 4 h, not to exceed 6 tabs a day
Vicodin 5 mg/300 mg	Hydrocodone and acetaminophen	Hydrocodone 5 mg and acetaminophen 300 mg	One tab every 4–6 h, not to exceed 8 tabs a day
Vicodin ES 7.5 mg/300 mg	Hydrocodone and acetaminophen	Hydrocodone 7.5 mg and acetaminophen 300 mg	One tab every 4–6 h, not to exceed 6 tabs a day
Loratab 5 mg or 7.5 mg	Hydrocodone and acetaminophen	Hydrocodone 5 mg or 7.5 mg and acetaminophen 500 mg	One tab every 4–6 h, not to exceed 8 tabs a day

B Severe Pain Management

Drug name	Ingredients	Doses	Directions
Vicodin HP 10 mg/300 mg	Hydrocodone and acetaminophen	Hydrocodone 10 mg and acetaminophen 300 mg	One tablet every 4–6 h, not to exceed 6 tabs a day
Oxycodone 5 mg	Oxycodone	5 mg	One tab every 4–6 h, not to exceed 6 tabs a day
Percocet	Oxycodone and acetaminophen	Oxycodone 2.5, 5, 7.5 or 10 mg and acetaminophen 325 mg	One tab every 4–6 h, not to exceed 6 tabs a day

(continued)

Drug name	Ingredients	Doses	Directions
Tylox	Oxycodone and acetaminophen	Oxycodone 5 mg and acetaminophen 500 mg	One tab every 4–6 h, not to exceed 6 tabs a day
Dilaudid	Hydromorphone	2, 4, or 8 mg	One tab every 4 h
Demerol	Mepridine	50 or 100 mg	One tab every 4 h

2 Antibacterial Infection

Drug name	Ingredient	Dose	Directions
Amoxicillin 500 mg	Amoxicillin	500 mg	One tab three times a day
Augmentin	Amoxicillin trihydrate 250, 500, or 875 mg plus clavulanate potassium 125 mg	250, 500, or 875 mg	One tab three times a day for 250 and 500 mg; one tab twice a day for 875 mg
Keflex	Cephalexin	250, 500, or 750 mg	One tab four times a day
Cleocin	Clindamycin	300 mg	One tab four times a day
Zithromycin	Azithromycin	500 mg	One tab every day for three days (for sinus infection)
Levaquin	Levofloxacin	250 or 500 mg	One tab a day for 10 days

3 Sinus Bacterial Infection

Bacteria responsible for allograft infections	Premedication prior to maxillary sinus augmentation	Infection
Staphylococcus aureus Viridans streptococci *Bacteroides*	Levaquin: 500 mg 1 h before procedure, then once daily for 10 days	Occurs in 3% of sinus graft cases 3 days after surgery.
	Amoxicillin: 500 mg or 1 gm 1 h before procedure, then three times daily (TID) for 7 days	Extend antibiotic coverage. Consider culture.
	Cephalosporin (Cefaclor): 500 mg or 1 gm 1 h before procedure, then four times daily (QID) for 7 days	

Bacteria responsible for allograft infections	Premedication prior to maxillary sinus augmentation	Infection
	Clindamycin (Cleocin): 150 mg or 300 mg 1 h before procedure, then TID for 7 days	

4 Xerostomia[2,3]

Etiology

- ◉ Medications
- ◉ Nerve damage (head and neck); no signal to the glands
- ◉ Sjögren's syndrome
- ◉ Diabetes
- ◉ HIV
- ◉ Smoking, alcohol, and/or caffeine
- ◉ Radiation treatment
- ◉ Cancer of the salivary glands
- ◉ Connective tissue disease
- ◉ Rheumatoid arthritis
- ◉ Systemic lupus erythematosus
- ◉ Systemic sclerosis
- ◉ Mixed connective tissue disease
- ◉ Primary biliary cirrhosis
- ◉ Vasculitis
- ◉ Chronic active hepatitis
- ◉ Bone marrow transplantation
- ◉ Renal dialysis
- ◉ Anxiety or depression

A   Drugs Associated with Xerostomia

Analgesic agents (central nervous system opioids)	Anorexiants
	Antihistaminic agents
Nonsteroidal anti-inflammatory drugs	Diuretic agents
Antihypertensive agents	Muscle relaxant agents
Sedatives and anxiolytic agents	Smoking cessation agents
Anticonvulsant agents	Bronchial dilator agents
Antiparkinsonian agents	Ophthalmic formulations

B   Clinical Manifestations of Xerostomia

Dry mouth and dry eyes Oral burning or soreness, or a sensation of a loss of or altered taste	Increased need to sip or drink water when swallowing Difficulty with swallowing dry foods Progressive parotid gland enlargement

Diagnosis	Management

Diagnosis

◉ Patient Interview

 Does your mouth usually feel dry?

 Does your mouth feel dry when eating a meal?

 Do you have difficulty swallowing dry foods?

 Do you sip liquids to aid in swallowing dry foods?

 Is the amount of saliva in your mouth too little most of the time?

◉ Salivary output test (less than 0.12 to 0.16 mm per minute unstimulated).

◉ Sialography and scintigraphy to measure salivary glands' function.

◉ Clinical laboratory abnormalities (Sjögren's syndrome) may disclose anemia, leukopenia, an increased erythrocyte sedimentation rate, and the presence of rheumatoid factor or autoantibodies.

◉ Biopsy from the lower lip may reveal focal lymphocytic infiltrates in the minor salivary glands.

Management

◉ If the patient's xerostomia is caused by the side effect of a drug, the dentist can recommend an alternative medication or *modification of dosage.*

◉ Avoid the use of alcoholic beverages and mouth rinses. Mouth rinses containing alcohol may desiccate the oral mucosa and worsen xerostomic symptoms.

◉ Use a humidifier at night.

◉ Use salivary flow stimulants such as:

 – sugarless chewing gum
 – Biotène rinse
 – sugarless hard candies

Saliva Substitutes and Oral Lubricants

◉ Moi-Stir (Kingswood Laboratories, Indianapolis, IN)

◉ MouthKote (Parnell Pharmaceuticals, Larkspur, CA)

◉ ORALbalance (Laclede, Rancho Dominguez, CA)

◉ Salivart (Xenex Laboratories, Coquitlam, BC, Canada)

◉ Xero-Lube (Colgate Oral Pharmaceuticals, Canton, MA)

Cholinergic Drugs

Parasympathomimetic stimulating agents:

◉ Cevimeline (Evoxac, Daiichi Pharmaceutical, Montvale, NJ)

◉ Pilocarpine (Salagen, MGI Pharma, Minneapolis, MN), 5–10 mg 3–4 times per day

5 Recommendations

Symptoms	Recommendations
⊛ Denture discomfort accompanied by loss of retention. ⊛ Susceptibility to infection of the oral cavity and oropharynx by the opportunistic fungus *Candida albicans*.	⊛ Avoid implants supported by a removable prosthesis. ⊛ Monitor for periodic use of antiviral or antimicrobial medications.

References

1 Pirie S. Surgical gowning and gloving. J Perioper Pract 2010 Jun;20(6):207–209.
2 A mandibular implant-supported fixed complete dental prosthesis in a patient with Sjögren syndrome: case report. Implant Dent 2010 Jun;19(3):178–183.
3 Thirteen-year follow-up of a mandibular implant-supported fixed complete denture in a patient with Sjögren's syndrome: a clinical report. J Prosthet Dent 2005 Nov;94(5):409–413.

3

Surgical Treatment

Part A: Immediate Implants

1 Classification[1]

	Type 1 Immediate	Type 2 Early placement: soft tissue healing	Type 3 Early placement with partial bone healing	Type 4 Late placement
Definition	– Immediate placement after tooth extraction – Considered part of the same procedure	– 4–8 weeks post extraction – Complete soft tissue coverage has occurred.	– 12–16 weeks post extraction – Substantial clinical and radio-graphical bone fill of the socket	– 16 weeks or more post extraction – Complete bone fill of the socket
Advantages	• Reduced surgical procedures • Reduced overall treatment times	• Reduced treatment time • Additional soft tissue volume allows for tension-free closure.	• Easier primary stability • Soft tissue volume allows for tension-free closure. • Peri-implant defects are 2–3 walled (favorable).	• Easy initial stability • Soft tissue volume allows for tension-free closure. • Soft tissue volume allows for better esthetic outcome.

Quick Reference to Dental Implant Surgery, First Edition. Mohamed A. Maksoud.
© 2017 John Wiley & Sons, Inc. Published 2017 by John Wiley & Sons, Inc.

	Type 1 Immediate	Type 2 Early placement: soft tissue healing	Type 3 Early placement with partial bone healing	Type 4 Late placement
	• Peri-implant defects are 2 or 3 walled, which is favorable for simultaneous bone augmentation procedures.	• Additional soft tissue allows for better esthetic outcome. • Peri-implant defects present are 2–3 walled (favorable). • Allows for resolution of pathology with extracted tooth	• Allows for resolution of pathology • Flattening of bone surface allows for easy grafting of the site.	• Allows for resolution of pathology
Disadvantages	• Difficult positioning • Difficult initial stability • Difficult primary closure due to reduced soft tissue volume • Increased risk of recession • Inability to predict bone remodeling	• Two surgical procedures required • Compromised initial stability	• Two surgical procedures • Extended treatment time • Socket wall has varying amounts of bone resorption. • Increased horizontal bone loss (limited bone available for implant placement)	• Two surgical procedures • Extended treatment time • Socket walls exhibit the greatest amount of resorption. • Greatest amount of bone loss

A   Case Selection

1. An extraction site with little or no bone loss
2. Sufficient bone height
3. Sufficient bone width
4. Sufficient buccal bone and adequate gingival biotype
5. Minimal circumferential defects
6. No pathology

B   Posterior Immediate Implants[2]

Posterior immediate implants can be considered challenging due to the following reasons:

– Incompatibility of extraction socket shape with commercially available implant shapes.
– Possibility of loss of remaining socket walls.
– Number of extraction sockets.

2   Procedure

❖ Extraction (atraumatic)
❖ Implant selection (select an implant longer than the extracted tooth by at least 3 mm)
❖ Place subcrestal 2–4 mm in anticipation for post-extraction vertical bone loss.

❖ 0.5 mm of crestal bone remodeling upon loading of the crown (Berglundh and Lindhe 1992 animal study). It continues from 0.5 mm to an area of high density until it stops (Misch 1995).
❖ Bone graft with or without membrane

3   General Advantages and Disadvantages

Advantages	Disadvantages
❖ Reduces surgical time	❖ Requires skillful operator
❖ Preserves bone level	❖ Bone graft and membrane
❖ Esthetics	

4 Complications[3] and Treatment

Complications	Treatment
❖ Infection	❖ Remove implant, graft, and replace implant.
❖ Nerve damage	❖ Monitor patient or remove implant.
❖ Iatrogenic damage to neighboring teeth	❖ Monitor patient or remove implant.
❖ Interproximal bone loss and black triangle	❖ Gingival augmentation Surgical foil and glue
❖ Lack of primary wound closure	❖ Gingival graft
❖ Need for gingival augmentation following or at the time of exposure	

5 Immediate Loading

Why?	Why not?
Better emergence profile	Possibility of failure
Preserve interdental papilla	More chair time to fabricate temporary
Faster healing	Could be costlier in the long run
Accelerate treatment	
Better esthetics	

6 Immediate Loading: When To?

Initial stability: if initial implant stability is achieved with 35 newton centimeters of torque No major bone grafting	No heavy overjet and overbite No heavy protrusive interferences No parafunctional habits

7 Recommendations

The key to immediate implants placement is the preservation of the extraction socket walls.	Primary stability of the immediate implant is a crucial factor in implant survival.

Figures 3.1 through 3.8 show extraction of a maxillary central incisor followed by immediate implant placement and a provisional.

Figure 3.1 Clinical photo of fractured right maxillary central incisor.

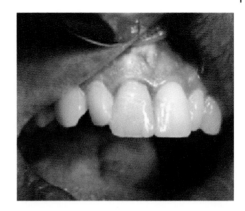

Figure 3.2 Radiograph of the same tooth.

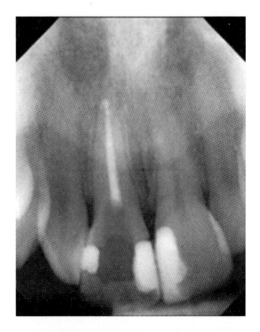

Figure 3.3 The extraction socket following atraumatic extraction.

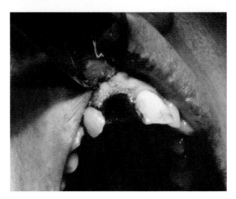

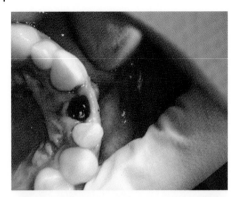

Figure 3.4 Immediate implant in place.

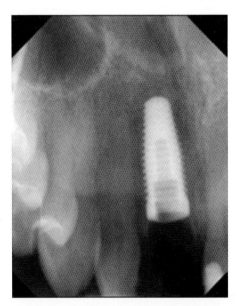

Figure 3.5 Radiograph of the implant in place.

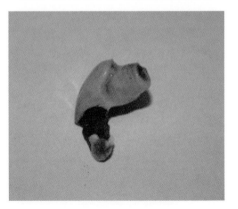

Figure 3.6 Resin-cemented provisional crown with sulcus former.

Figure 3.7 Radiograph of the provisional crown.

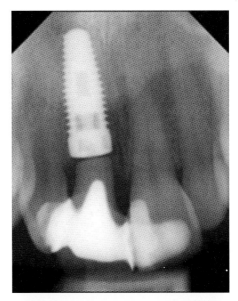

Figure 3.8 Clinical photo of the provisional crown.

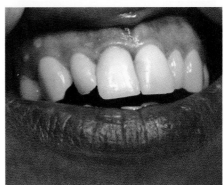

Part B: Sinus Augmentation

1 Maxillary Sinus Anatomy[4]

- Develops at age 3 months due to pressure from growth of eyes into the orbit
- Complete pneumatization at 16–18 years
- Further expansion as a result of posterior teeth loss

- Pyramid shape with 4 thin bony walls
- Base of pyramid toward the zygomatic process
- 34 × 35 mm at the base; apex extends 23 mm
- Volume 15 ml
- Underdeveloped in 8% of cases

2 Anatomical Considerations

Anterior wall	Posterior wall
Infra-orbital nerve and blood vessels run in that wall, which could be less than 10 mm from the crest of the extremely edentulous maxilla	Pterygomaxillary region
	Has the posterior superior alveolar nerve and blood vessels
	Has the interior maxillary artery
Superior wall	AVOID contact with the posterior wall due to possible bleeding and nerve damage.
Orbital floor. Dehiscence in that wall can result in direct contact with the sinus mucosa.	
	Medial wall
AVOID contact with the anterior wall due to the possible complications of diplopia (affecting vision).	Supports the lower and middle conchae
	Maxillary ostium (the main drainage pipe of the sinus)
Floor wall	Sinus membrane
Maxillary posterior teeth	Floor: mucoperiosteal
Lateral wall	All other: mucous membrane
Zygomatic process	

A Blood Supply and Drainage

Arterial blood supply of the sinus	Medial wall to the nasopalatine vein (15% of brain abscess)
Ethmoid artery	
Branches from nasal mucosa	All other walls drain to pterygomaxillary plexus.
Branches from infraorbital, facial, and palatine arteries	
	Lymphatic drainage
Venous drainage	Drain to the middle meatus mucosal lymph nodes.

B Physical Exam

- Polyps in the nostrils
- Cystic lesions in the nostrils
- Neoplasm (60% of squamous cell carcinoma of the paranasal sinuses)
- Cocaine abuse is reflected in redness of the nasal mucosa.
- Oro-antral fistula

3 Procedure Steps

Figures 3.9 through 3.15 illustrate an open maxillary left sinus augmentation procedure with a window osteotomy, membrane elevation, and bone augmentation.

A   Postoperative Instructions

- Do not blow your nose.
- No flying, diving, or waterskiing for 6 weeks.
- Sleep with two pillows behind your neck.
- Do not use a straw for drinking.
- Do not smoke.
- Do not lower your head.
- Do not sneeze.

Figure 3.9 Clinical photo of the edentulous space maxillary left area.

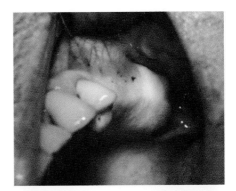

Figure 3.10 The window osteotomy.

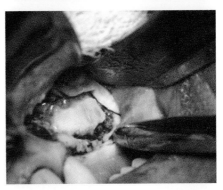

Figure 3.11 Window elevated.

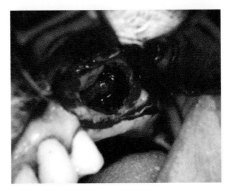

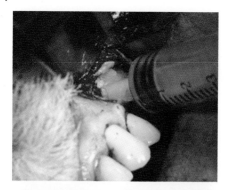

Figure 3.12 Bone graft putty injected into the created window space.

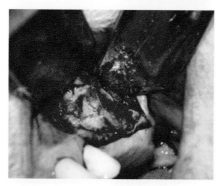

Figure 3.13 Complete packing of the bone graft.

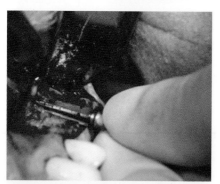

Figure 3.14 An implant bone drill held to determine adequate bone height for the proposed implant.

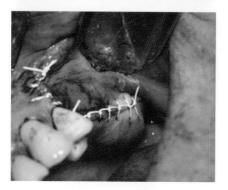

Figure 3.15 Mattress suture of the surgical area, including the horizontal and vertical incisions.

Perioperative	Membrane perforation	Postoperative short-term complications	Postoperative long-term complications
• *Bleeding*: use bone wax and vasoconstrictors.	• *Minor membrane perforation*: use fast-absorbing collagen membrane. • *Moderate membrane perforation*: fold membrane over tear by continuing elevation on opposite corners. Use slow-resorbing collagen membrane. May need to delay implant placement. • *Large perforation*: abort procedure.	• *Incision line opening*: occurs due to lateral ridge augmentation. • *Crestal opening*: leave to granulate. • *Vertical incision opening*: surgical glue or resuture after undermining the buccal flap to release tension. • *Infection*: occurs in 3% of sinus graft cases 3 days after surgery. Extend antibiotic coverage; consider culture.	• Mucocele formation • Chronic sinusitis • Loss of graft materials and failure of implant • Overpacking and obliteration of the sinus • Orbital cellulites • Optic neuritis • Cavernous sinus thrombosis • Epidural and subdural infection • Meningitis • Cerebritis • Blindness • Osteomylitis • Consult with medical professionals for treatment

Part C: Ridge Augmentation

1   Soft Tissue Augmentation

Soft tissue gingival augmentation is commonly rendered in edentulous spaces for the purpose of filling gaps underneath the fixed prosthesis pontic in order to maximize esthetics. The following is an example of the augmentation procedure utilizing an acellular dermal matrix. Figures 3.16 through 3.23 show soft tissue augmentation underneath the left maxillary canine pontic using an allograft.

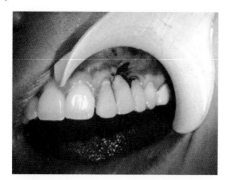

Figure 3.16 Preoperative.

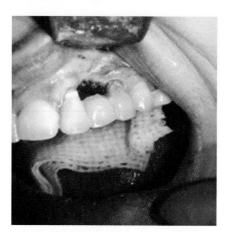

Figure 3.17 Shortening the pontic to allow for the implanted tissue.

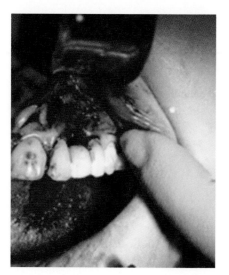

Figure 3.18 Tunnel vertical incision, full thickness.

Figure 3.19 The dermal acellular matrix folded to increase the volume.

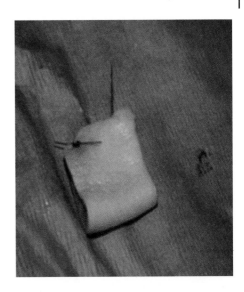

Figure 3.20 The matrix implanted.

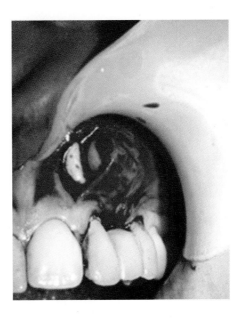

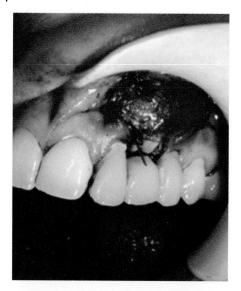

Figure 3.21 Postoperative healing.

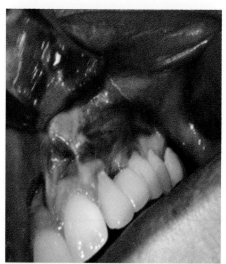

Figure 3.22 Postoperative healing.

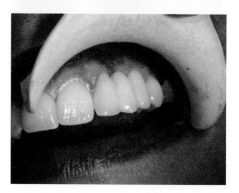

Figure 3.23 Complete healing with adequate soft tissue augmentation below the pontic.

2 Onlay Grafts[5]

	Symphysis	Ramus	Tuberosity
Surgical access	Good	Fair to good	Good to fair
Patient cosmetic concern	High	High	Low
Graft shape	Thick block	Thin veneer	Porous block
Graft size	≥1 cm	≤1 cm	≤1 cm
Graft resorption	Minimal	Moderate	Moderate
Healed bone quality	D1 D2	D1 D2	D3
Postoperative pain and edema	Moderate	Minimal	Minimal
Nerve damage, teeth	Common	Uncommon	Uncommon
Nerve damage, soft tissue	Common	Common	Uncommon
Incision dehiscence	Occasional	Uncommon	Uncommon
Sinus perforation	None	None	Occasional

3 Titanium Straps, Cores, and Screws

Figures 3.24 through 3.33 illustrate augmentation of an atrophic premaxilla using a mandibular mental block graft, core grafts, titanium straps, and screws.

Figure 3.24 Donor site of mental graft.

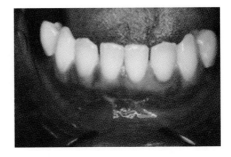

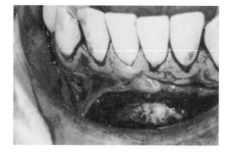

Figure 3.25 Bone harvesting from donor site.

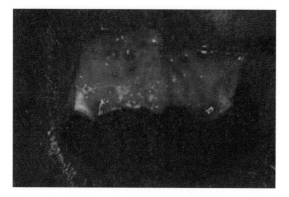

Figure 3.26 Premaxillary ridge deficiency.

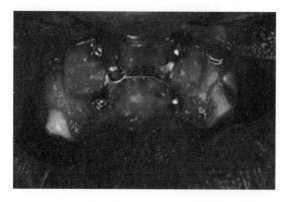

Figure 3.27 Mental onlay grafts in recipient site secured with titanium straps.

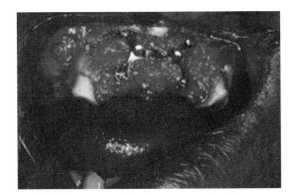

Figure 3.28 Voids between only graft and recipient site are filled with allograft particulates.

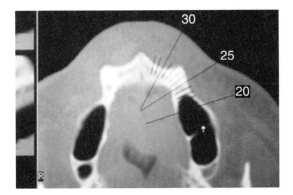

Figure 3.29 CT scan of the premaxillary defect prior to the augmentation.

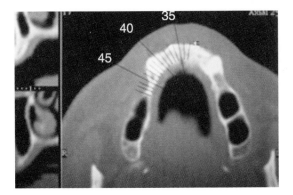

Figure 3.30 CT scan of the premaxillary defect following the augmentation.

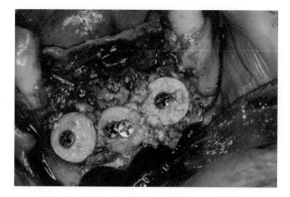

Figure 3.31 Onlay grafts harvested below the atrophic site and secured in place with titanium screws.

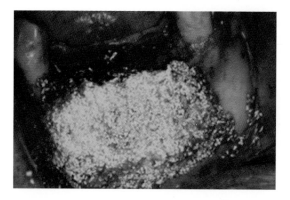

Figure 3.32 The recipient site and the onlay graft covered with particulate allograft.

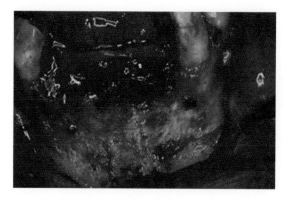

Figure 3.33 Healed recipient and donor sites.

4   Titanium Mesh, Distraction Osteogenesis, J Block, and Ridge Expansion

	Titanium mesh	Distraction osteogenesis	J block	Ridge expansion
Advantages	Predictable	Little relapse Bigger movements possible Outpatient surgery Generation of soft tissue Less likelihood of nerve injury	Suitable for large deficiency Allograft; no morbidity	Eliminates the need for bone graft Condenses cancellous bone for maximizing osseo-integration
Disadvantages	Need for second surgery to remove mesh Possible exposure of the mesh and tissue necrosis	Technique-sensitive surgery Equipment-sensitive surgery Possible need of second surgery to remove distraction devices Patient compliance	High risk of necrosis due to lack of blood supply Requires surgical training	Risk of bone separation Mallet use with the bone spreader could be unacceptable to patients.

5   Membranes

❖ Biocompatible
❖ Easy to cut
❖ Mechanically stiff for space making
❖ No or low memory
❖ If resorbable, not to interfere with osteogenesis
❖ *Space maintenance*
❖ *Predictability of results: functions as a barrier during the critical period of wound healing*
❖ *Absorbable*
❖ *Cell-occlusive: prevents epithelial cell migration*
❖ *Wound stabilization: helps stabilize and maintain blood clot in the defect space*

Defect	Recommendation
Less than 3 mm horizontal	Particulate cortico-cancellous demineralized allograft with resorbable membrane
Less than 3 mm vertical	Place implant supracrestal, and build bone around it using the same bone source and membrane.
More than 3 mm horizontal	Autogenous block graft from the chin, ascending ramus, and tuberosity
More than 3 mm vertical	Titanium mesh with autologous graft or stem cell allograft
More than 6 mm vertical or horizontal	Titanium mesh with allograft

Part D: Extraction Socket Preservation

1 Advantages

❖ Alveolar ridge dimensions are preserved, also in non-implant restorations (pontic areas in crown and bridge restorations).[1]
❖ Optimal esthetics of the teeth and soft tissue can be achieved, even in challenging regions.
❖ Therapeutic window for implant placement is extended.
❖ Extent of future invasive surgery can be reduced.
❖ No second-stage surgery
❖ Less trauma (psychological and physical)
❖ Decrease in postoperative complications
❖ Time savings
❖ Decrease in cost of future grafting
❖ Maintain ridge height and width.
❖ Fulfill patient's demand for ideal aesthetic outcome.
❖ Reduce treatment time.
❖ Avoid complex augmentation procedures in cases with severe resorption of the buccal bone crest.
❖ Achieve an optimal soft tissue healing before implant placement.
❖ Create a favorable situation for early implant placement in the ideal prosthetic position.
❖ Increase buccal contour, and reduce or avoid soft tissue grafting.
❖ Achieve optimal clinical results.

2 Steps for Good Extraction Socket Development

1. Intrasulcular incision
2. Minimal flap elevation
3. Preserve buccal wall.
4. Section endodontically treated or fractured tooth first
5. Extract.
6. Degranulate socket.
7. If no spontaneous bleeding, initiate it by a bur.
8. Graft.
9. Membrane (tuck 3–4 mm under flaps)
10. Freshen epithelial flap edges.
11. Undermine buccal flap for tension free.
12. Suture removal: 2 weeks
13. Membrane removal: 4–6 weeks
14. Implant: 3–6 months
15. Full maturation: 12–18 weeks

3 Complications

Complication	Recommendation
Membrane exposure, partial	Chlorhexidine mouthwash, antibiotics, resuturing, or surgical glue.
Membrane exposure, major	Consider removing the membrane if non-resorbable.
Drainage and infection, minor	Antibiotics; reassess in two weeks
Drainage and infection, major	Remove bone and membrane; broad-spectrum antibiotics.

4 Recommendations

Intact buccal plate, anterior tooth	Bone graft with or without a membrane
Intact buccal plate, posterior tooth	Bone graft with a resorbable membrane
Partial loss of buccal plate	Bone graft with a resorbable membrane covering the buccal defect and bone mass
Complete loss of buccal plate	Buccal full-thickness flap with vertical releasing incision. Bone graft with delayed resorbable or non-resorbable membrane

Part E: Suture Materials[6]

1 Monofilament and Multifilament Sutures

Monofilament	Multifilament
• Monofilament suture made of a single strand • Less resistant to harboring microorganisms • Less resistance to passage through tissue than multifilament suture • Great care must be taken in handling and tying monofilament suture because crushing or crimping of this suture can nick or *weaken* the suture and lead to undesirable and premature suture failure.	• Multifilament suture composed of several filaments twisted or braided together • Less stiff but have a higher coefficient of friction • Greater tensile strength and better pliability and flexibility than monofilament suture • Due to the increased capillarity, the increased absorption of fluid may act as a tract for the introduction of pathogens.
Absorbable	Non-absorbable
• Absorbable sutures provide temporary wound support, until the wound heals well enough to withstand normal stress. • Absorption occurs by enzymatic *degradation* in *natural materials* and by *hydrolysis* in *synthetic materials*. Hydrolysis causes less tissue reaction than enzymatic degradation. • The first stage of absorption lasts for several days to weeks. • The second stage is characterized by loss of suture mass and overlaps the first stage. • Loss of suture mass occurs as a result of leukocytic cellular responses that remove cellular debris and suture material from the line of tissue approximation. • Chemical treatments, such as chromic salts, lengthen the absorption time.	• Non-absorbable sutures elicit a tissue reaction that results in encapsulation of the suture material by fibroblasts. • The US Pharmacopeia classification is as follows: Class I: Silk or synthetic fibers of monofilament, twisted, or braided construction Class II: Cotton or linen fibers or coated natural or synthetic fibers in which the coating contributes to suture thickness without adding strength Class III: Metal wire of monofilament or multifilament construction

2   Absorbable and Non-absorbable Sutures

Natural	Synthetic
Plain Gut • Tensile strength is maintained for 7–10 days; absorption is complete within 70 days. Used for: • For repairing rapidly healing tissues that require minimal support • Also for ligating superficial blood vessels. *Chromic Gut (Treated with Chromium Salt)* • Tensile strength is maintained for 10–14 days. The absorption rate is slowed by chromium salt. • Have a tendency to fray during knot construction	• Polyglactin (Vicryl) • Poliglecaprone 25 (Monocryl) • Polysorb • Polydioxanone (PDS II) • Caprosyn • Polytrimethylene carbonate (Maxon)

3   Natural and Synthetic Sutures

Natural	Synthetic
• Surgical silk • Surgical cotton • Surgical steel	• Nylon • Monofilament (Ethilon and Monosof) • Braided (Nurolon and Surgilon) • Polyester fiber (Mersilene and Surgidac) • Polybutester suture (Novafil) • Coated polybutester suture (Vascufil) • Polypropylene (Prolene) • Surgipro II • PTFE

4 Recommendations

A Periodontal Surgery

Suture type	Construction	Strength retention profile	Absorption profile	Other
Plain gut	Monofilament	7–10 days	70 days	Tensile strength for 10–14 days
Chromic gut	Monofilament	21–28 days	70 days	Tensile strength for 10–14 days
Vicryl Rapide	Braided	75% at 14 days 50% at 21 days 25% at 4 weeks 50% at 5 days 0% at 10–14 days	42–70 days 42 days	High tissue inflammation Good knot security
Monocryl	Monofilament	50% at 7 days 20% at 14 days	91–119 days	Ease of handling
PDS	Monofilament	60% at 14 days 40% at 4 weeks 25% at 6 weeks	183–238 days	Low tensile strength
Polysorb	Braided	80% at 14 days 30% at 21 days	56–70 days	Wound support for 3 weeks only
Maxon	Monofilament	70% at 14 days 25% at 42 days	180 days	Wound support for 6 weeks
Dexon	Braided	75% at 14 days 50% at 21 days 25% at 4 weeks	42–70 days	Wound support for 3 weeks
Caprosyn	Monofilament	50% at 5 days 20% at 10 days 0% at 21 days	60–90 days	Wound support for 10 days
Biosyn	Monofilament	75% at 14 days 40% at 21 days	90–110 days	Wound support for 3 weeks

B   Implant and Bone Surgery

Suture	Type	Strength retention profile
Ethilon	Monofilament	81% for one year
Nurolon	Braided	81% for one year
Novafill	Monofilament	Has elasticity feature when stretched
Mersilene	Braided	100% for 1 year
Prolene	Monofilament	100% for 2 years
Surgipro	Braided	100% for 2 years
PTFE	Monofilament	
Silk	Braided	100% for 1 year
Ethibond	Braided	100%

References

1 Hammerle CH, Chen ST, Wilson TG Jr. Consensus statements and recommended clinical procedures regarding the placement of implants in extraction sockets. Int J Oral Maxillofac Implants 2004;19(suppl):26–28.

2 Maksoud MA. Immediate implants in fresh posterior extraction sockets: report of two cases. J Oral Implantol 2001;27(3):123–126.

3 Fugazzotto PA. Maxillary sinus grafting with and without simultaneous implant placement: technical consideration and clinical reports. Int J Periodontics Restorative Dent 1994;14:545–551.

4 Chen ST, Darby IB, Reynolds EC. A prospective clinical study of nonsubmerged immediate implants: clinical outcomes and esthetic results. Clin Oral Implants Res 2007;18:552–562.

5 Kuchler U, von Arx T. Horizontal ridge augmentation in conjunction with or prior to implant placement in the anterior maxilla: a systematic review. Proceedings of the Difth ITI Consensus Conference 2014;(suppl 5).

6 Maksoud M, Koo S, Barouch K, Karimbux N. Popularity of suture materials among residents and faculty members of a postdoctoral periodontology program. J Inves Clin Dent 2013;4:1–6.

4

Corrective Implant Surgery

Part A: Clinical Recommendations for the Prevention and Treatment of Peri-implant Disease[1]

Peri-implant health	Peri-implant mucositis	Peri-implantitis
Diagnosis Absence of clinical signs of inflammation.	*Diagnosis* Presence of individual clinical signs of soft tissue inflammation (e.g., redness, edema, and suppuration) and bleeding on gentle probing.	*Diagnosis* Presence of mucositis in conjunction with progressive crestal bone loss.
Treatment A recall frequency of at least once per year is recommended unless systemic and/or local conditions require more frequent intervals. In cases of peri-implant health, professional cleaning including reinforcement of self-performed oral hygiene is recommended as a preventive measure.	*Treatment* Reinforcement of self-performed oral hygiene. Mechanical debridement with or without antiseptics (e.g., chlorhexidine). The use of systemic antibiotics for the treatment of peri-implant mucositis is not justified. Therapy of peri-implant mucositis should be considered as a preventive measure for the onset of peri-implantitis.	*Treatment* Early implementation of appropriate therapy is recommended to prevent further progression of the disease. See Part B, "Peri-implantitis Treatment Recommendations."

Quick Reference to Dental Implant Surgery, First Edition. Mohamed A. Maksoud.
© 2017 John Wiley & Sons, Inc. Published 2017 by John Wiley & Sons, Inc.

Part B: Peri-implantitis Treatment Recommendations[2,3]

Presurgical	Nonsurgical	Surgical	Postsurgical
1. Thorough assessment and diagnosis. 2. Reduction of risk factors for peri-implantitis, in particular poor oral hygiene, prostheses that prevent adequate access for plaque control, tobacco use, the presence of periodontal diseases, and systemic diseases that may predispose to peri-implant disease. 3. If required, prosthesis removal and adjustment/replacement.	Debridement focused on maximal removal of biofilm, with or without antimicrobials.	1. Full-thickness mucoperiosteal flaps and removal of granulation tissue to allow thorough cleaning of the implant surface. 2. For thorough surface decontamination of the implant and restorative components, the following techniques have been proposed: locally applied chemicals like citric acid, tetracycline, and EDTA; gauze soaked with saline or antiseptics; hand-powered instruments; air-powder abrasives; Er-YAG lasers; photodynamic therapy; and implant surface modification. 3. Surgical therapy might also include regenerative or resective approaches.	1. The immediate postoperative anti-infective protocol should include daily chlorhexidine rinsing during the healing period until mechanical oral hygiene can be resumed. 2. Antibiotics are recommended in view of the aggressive nature of disease. 3. Professional support of cleaning and plaque control will be needed during this phase. 4. Clinical monitoring should be performed on a regular basis and supplemented by appropriate radiographic evaluation as required.

4. Regenerative approaches include filling of the intraosseous peri-implant defect with a bone substitute, graft, or bioactive substance with or without a resorbable barrier membrane. Submerged healing might reduce the risk of membrane exposure.

5. Resective approaches include osseous recontouring with apical positioning of the flap.

6. The clinician should consider implant removal as a treatment option. Factors influencing this decision may include the severity of the peri-implantitis lesion, the position of the implant, the surrounding tissues, or when the treatment outcomes are likely to be unsatisfactory.

7. Referral to specialist care for nonresponding peri-implantitis should be considered.

Supportive

5. Maintenance therapy, including reinforcement of effective oral hygiene and professional biofilm removal, should be provided on a frequency determined by oral health and the risk profile, likely to be every 3 to 6 months.

6. The patient should be advised that:

a. Recession of the peri-implant mucosa should be expected following peri-implantitis treatment, in particular after surgical therapy.

b. Progression or recurrence of disease might require additional therapy or implant removal.

Case 1, in Figures 4.1 through 4.5, illustrates peri-implantitis of mandibular posterior implants with moderate bone loss on the buccal aspect. Treatment consisted of autogenous graft harvested from the mandible and covered with a membrane.

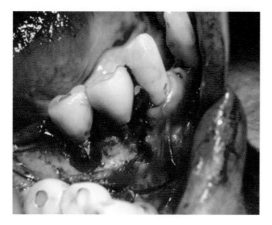

Figure 4.1 Case 1: moderate peri-implantitis.

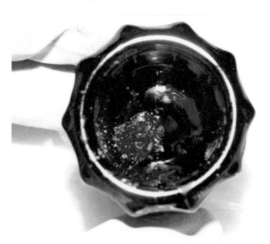

Figure 4.2 Autogenous bone harvested.

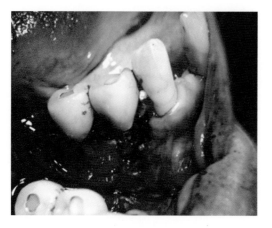

Figure 4.3 Grafted implant surface after surface treatment.

Figure 4.4 Resorbable membrane covering the bone graft.

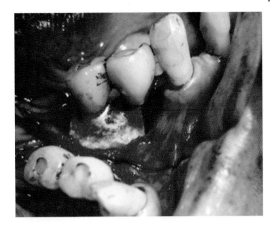

Figure 4.5 Flap sutured to ensure complete coverage of the bone graft and membrane.

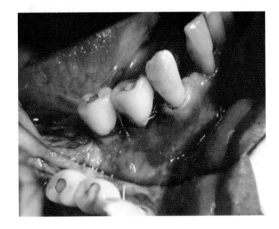

Case 2, in Figures 4.6 through 4.12, shows peri-implantitis of maxillary posterior implant with severe bone loss. The treatment of choice was to remove the implant via a trephine drill followed by immediate implant placement, bone augmentation and a membrane.

Figure 4.6 Case 2: severe peri-implantitis.

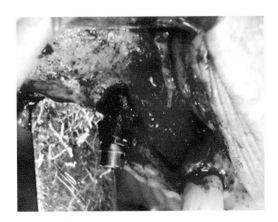

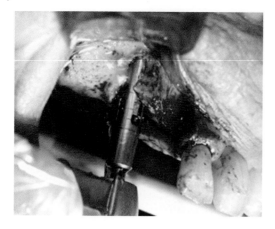

Figure 4.7 Trephine drill used to remove implant.

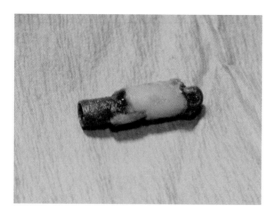

Figure 4.8 Removed implant.

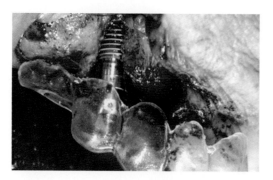

Figure 4.9 New implant placed using surgical stent.

Figure 4.10 Bone graft to fill in the voids between the new implant and the walls of the osteotomy.

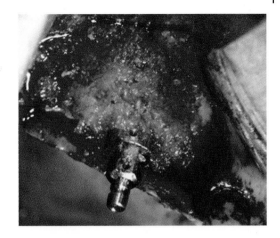

Figure 4.11 Membrane covering the bone graft.

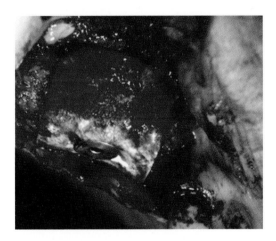

Figure 4.12 Sutured flap.

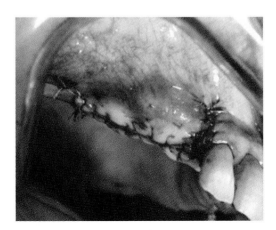

Case 3, in Figures 4.13 through 4.17, illustrates peri-implantitis due to trauma from an orthodontic appliance attempting to distalize the posterior molar that have resulted in bone separation from the implant surface. The treatment consisted of suspending the orthodontic treatment followed by bone augmentation and a membrane.

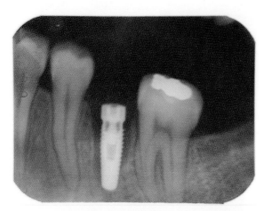

Figure 4.13 Case 3: peri-implantitis due to trauma from orthodontic appliance.

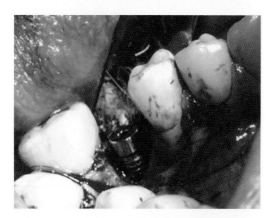

Figure 4.14 Implant surface cleaned.

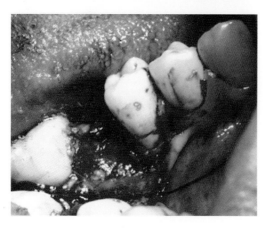

Figure 4.15 Grafted implant bone defect.

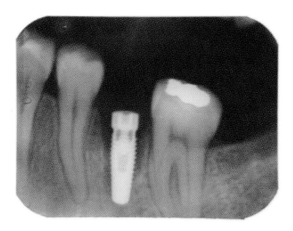

Figure 4.16 Radiograph before treatment.

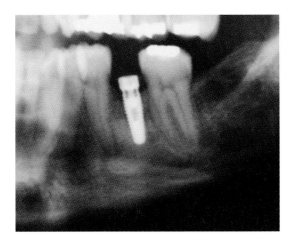

Figure 4.17 Radiograph after treatment.

References

1 Heitz-Mayfield LA, Needleman I, Salvi GE, Pjetursson BE. Consensus Statements and Clinical Recommendations for Prevention and Management of Biologic and Technical Implant Complications. Proceedings of the Fifth ITI Conference, 2014; 29:346–350.

2 Mombelli A, Müller N, Cionca N. The epidemiology of periimplantitis. Clin Oral Implants Res 2012; 23(suppl 6):67–76.

3 Heitz-Mayfield LJA, Salvi GE, Mombelli A, Faddy M, Lang NP, Implant Complication Research G. Anti-infective surgical therapy of periimplantitis. A 12-month prospective clinical study. Clin Oral Implants Res 2012; 23:205–210.

5

Errors and Complications

Part A: Diagnosis of Complications[1]

Host related	Material or design related	Practitioner or technique related	Unknown
1. Allergies to titanium	1. Implant fixture design and surface	1. Surgical errors	Complications due to unidentified reasons
2. Systemic conditions	2. Implant restoration design	2. Prosthetic errors	
3. Poor oral hygiene		3. Lack of maintenance protocol	
4. Uncontrolled or recurrent periodontal disease			
5. Smoking			
6. Parafunctional habits			
7. Lack of dental implant education			

Part B: Surgical Errors

1 Early Implant Failure

1. Dull surgical drills
2. Slow or excessive drilling speed
3. Over-torqueing of the implant
4. Inadequate irrigation during drilling

Quick Reference to Dental Implant Surgery, First Edition. Mohamed A. Maksoud.
© 2017 John Wiley & Sons, Inc. Published 2017 by John Wiley & Sons, Inc.

2 Late Implant Failure

1. Improper selection of implant diameter and length
2. Inadequate number of implants to support the prosthesis
3. Lack of identification of anatomical structures
4. Lack of identification of ridge defects
5. Improper soft tissue manipulation leading to recession

Part C: Prosthetic Errors

1. Lack of temporization in anterior implants
2. Unacceptable temporary prosthesis that results in damage to the soft tissue and bone surrounding the implants
3. Faulty restorations, open margins, and/or open contact
4. Excess cement around the implant
5. Gap between the implant fixture and prosthesis
6. Impingement from a temporary removable prosthesis

Part D: The Checklist

1 Basic Implant Placement[2]

✓ Update medical history and medications.
✓ Contact physician for discontinuation of blood thinners and for the use of epinephrine.
✓ Prescribe sedative and pre-medications as needed.
✓ Review computed tomography (CT) scan or film.
✓ Temporary removable prosthesis.
✓ Surgical stent.
✓ Select implant length and diameter.
✓ Bone graft material and membrane.
✓ Sign consent. Individual consents needed for multiple procedures.
✓ Administer anesthesia. Nerve blocks and infiltration.
✓ Create full-thickness mucoperiostal flaps, crestal and vertical if needed.
✓ Initial osteotomy.
✓ Take a radiograph to assess position, and correct if needed.
✓ Complete the osteotomy till the final diameter and length are achieved.
✓ Place implant.
✓ Place cover screw or healing abutment.
✓ Suture; allow for tension-free flap.
✓ Take final postoperative radiograph.

✓ Deliver temporary prosthesis.
✓ Postop instructions and ice pack.
✓ Medications.
✓ Schedule suture removal in 2 weeks.
✓ Next-day follow-up call.

References

1 Moneim A, Souza D. Avoiding Dental Implant Complications. Robertson, 2012.
2 Al-Faraje L. Oral Implantology Surgical Procedures Checklist. Quintessence, 2013.

6

Communication

Part A: Sample Consents

1 Endosseous Implant Consent

Consent form for Implant Placement and Anesthesia

Diagnosis. After an oral examination and study of my dental condition, my dentist has advised me that my missing tooth or teeth may be replaced with artificial teeth supported by an implant.

Recommended Treatment. In order to treat my condition, my dentist has recommended the use of root form dental implants. I understand that the procedure for root form implants involves placing implants into the jawbone. This procedure has a surgical phase followed by a prosthetic phase.

Surgical Phase of Procedure. I understand that sedation may be utilized and that a local anesthetic will be administered to me as part of the treatment. My gum tissue will be opened to expose the bone. Implants will be placed by tapping or threading them into holes that have been drilled in my jawbone. The implants will have to be snugly fitted and held tightly in place during the healing phase.

The gum and soft tissue will be stitched closed over or around the implants. A periodontal bandage or dressing may be placed. Healing will be allowed to proceed for a period of four to six months. I understand that dentures usually cannot be worn during the first one to two weeks of the healing phase.

I further understand that if clinical conditions turn out to be unfavorable for the use of this implant system or prevent the placement of implants, my dentist will make a professional judgment on the management of the situation. The procedure also may involve supplemental bone graft or other types of grafts to hold up the ridge of my jaw *and* thereby to assist in placement, closure, and security of my implants.

For implants requiring a second surgical procedure, the overlying tissues will be opened at the appropriate time, and the stability of the implant will be verified. If the implant appears satisfactory, an attachment will be connected to the implant. Plans and procedures to create an implant prosthetic appliance can then begin.

Quick Reference to Dental Implant Surgery, First Edition. Mohamed A. Maksoud.
© 2017 John Wiley & Sons, Inc. Published 2017 by John Wiley & Sons, Inc.

Prosthetic Phase of Procedure. I understand that at this point, I will be referred back to my dentist or to a prosthodontist. This phase is just as important as the surgical phase for the long-term success of the oral reconstruction. During this phase, an implant prosthetic device will be attached to the implant. This procedure should be performed by a person trained in the prosthetic protocol for the root form implant system.

Expected Benefits. The purpose of dental implants is to allow me to have more functional artificial teeth. The implants provide support, anchorage, and retention for these teeth.

Principal Risks and Complications. I understand that some patients do not respond successfully to dental implants, and in such cases, the implant may be lost. Implant surgery may not be successful in providing artificial teeth. Because each patient's condition is unique, long-term success may not occur.

I understand that complications may result from the implant surgery, drugs, and anesthetics.

These complications include, but are not limited to, postsurgical infection; bleeding; swelling and pain; facial discoloration; transient but on occasion permanent numbness of the lip, tongue, teeth, chin, or gum; jaw joint injuries or associated muscle spasm; transient but on occasion permanent increased tooth looseness; tooth sensitivity to hot, cold, sweet, or acidic foods; shrinkage of the gum upon healing, resulting in elongation of some teeth and greater spaces between some teeth; cracking or bruising of the corners of the mouth; restricted ability to open my mouth for several days or weeks; impact on well-being; allergic reactions; injury to teeth; bone fractures; nasal sinus penetrations; delayed healing; and accidental swallowing of foreign matter. The exact duration of any complications cannot be determined, and they may be irreversible.

I understand that the design and structure of the prosthetic appliance can be a substantial factor in the success or failure of the implant. I further understand that alterations made on the artificial appliance or the implant can lead to loss of the implant or appliance. This loss would be the sole responsibility of the person making such alterations. I am advised that the connection between the implant and the bone may fail and that it may become necessary to remove the implant. This can happen in the preliminary phase, during the initial integration of the implant to the bone, or at any time thereafter.

I understand that implant success is dependent upon a number of variables including, but *not* limited to: individual patient tolerance and health, anatomical variations, my home care of the implant, and habits such as grinding my teeth. I also understand that implants are available in a variety of designs and materials and the choice of implant is determined by the professional judgment of my dentist.

I have also been advised that there is a minimal risk that the implant may break, which may require additional procedures to repair or replace the broken implant.

Alternatives to Suggested Treatment. Alternative treatments for missing teeth include no treatment, new removable appliances, and other procedures – depending on the circumstances. However, continued wearing of ill-fitting and loose removable appliances can result in further damage to the bone and soft tissue of my mouth.

I have further been informed that if no treatment is elected to replace the missing teeth or existing dentures, the non-treatment risks include, but are not limited to:

(a) Maintenance of the existing full or partial denture(s), with relines or remakes every three to five years or as otherwise may be necessary due to slow but progressive dissolution of the underlying denture-supporting jawbone;
(b) Any present discomfort or chewing inefficiency with the existing partial or full denture may persist or worsen in time;
(c) Drifting, biting, and/or extrusion of remaining teeth;
(d) Looseness of teeth, periodontal disease (gum and bone), possibly followed by extraction(s); and
(e) A potential jaw joint problem caused by a deficient, collapsed, or otherwise improper bite.

Necessity Follow-up Care and Self-Care. I understand that it is important for me to continue to see my dentist or prosthodontist. Implants, natural teeth, and appliances have to be maintained daily in a clean, hygienic manner. Implants and appliances also must be examined periodically and may need to be adjusted.

I understand that it is important for me to abide by the specific prescriptions and instructions given by my dentist.

I promise to, and accept responsibility for failing to, return to this office for examinations and any recommended treatment, at least every six months. My failure to do so, for whatever reason, can jeopardize the clinical success of the implant system. I have been advised that smoking, alcohol, or sugar consumption may affect tissue healing and may limit the success of the implant. Because there is no way to accurately predict the gum-healing and bone-healing capabilities of each patient, I know I must follow my dentist's home care instructions and report to my dentist for regular examinations as instructed. I further understand that excellent home care, including brushing, flossing, and the use of any other device recommended by my dentist, is critical to the success of my treatment,and my failure to do what I am supposed to do at home will more than likely contribute to the failure of the implants.

Accordingly, I agree to release and hold my dentist harmless if my implant(s) fail as a result of not maintaining an ongoing examination and preventive maintenance routine as directed by my dentist.

No Warranty or Guarantee. I hereby acknowledge that no guarantee, warranty, or assurance has been given to me that the proposed treatment will be successful; due to individual patient differences, a dentist cannot predict certainty of success. There exists the risk of case relapse, additional treatment, or worsening of my present condition, including the possible loss of certain teeth, despite the best of care.

I am aware that the practice of dentistry and dental surgery is not an exact science, and I acknowledge that no guarantees have been made to me concerning the success of my implant surgery, the associated treatment and procedures, or the postsurgical dental procedures. I am further aware that there is a risk that the implant placement may fail, through no one's fault, which then might require further corrective surgery associated with the removal. Such a failure and remedial procedures could also involve additional fees being assessed.

Publication of Records. I authorize photos, slides, x-rays, or any other viewing of my care and treatment during or after its completion to be used for the advancement of dentistry and for reimbursement purposes. My identity will not be revealed to the general public, however, without my permission.

I have been fully informed of the nature of root form implant surgery, the procedure to be utilized, the risks and benefits of the surgery, the alternative treatments available, and the necessity for follow-up and self-care. I have had an opportunity to ask any questions I may have in connection with the treatment and to discuss my concerns with my dentist. After thorough deliberation, I hereby consent to the performance of dental implant surgery as presented to me during consultation and in the treatment plan presentation as described in this document.

I also consent to the use of an alternative implant system or method if clinical conditions are found to be unfavorable for the use of the implant system that has been described to me. If clinical conditions prevent the placement of implant, I defer to my dentist's judgment on the management of that situation. I also give my permission to receive supplemental bone grafts to build up the ridge of my jaw and thereby to assist in placement, closure, and security of my implants.

To my knowledge, I have given an accurate report of my health history. I have also reported *any* past allergic or other reactions to drugs, food, insect bites, anesthetics, blood diseases, gum or skin reactions, abnormal bleeding, or any other condition relating to my physical or mental health or any problems experienced with any prior medical, dental, or other health care treatment on my medical history questionnaire. I understand that certain mental and/or emotional disorders may increase the risk of failure or contraindicate implant therapy and have therefore expressly circled either YES or NO to indicate whether or not I have had any past treatment or therapy of any kind or type for any mental or emotional condition.

I realize and understand that the purpose of this document is to evidence the fact that I am knowingly consenting to the implant procedures recommended by my dentist.

I agree that if I do not follow my dentist's recommendations and advice for postoperative care, my dentist may terminate the dentist–patient relationship, requiring me to seek treatment from another dentist. I realize that postoperative care and maintenance treatment is critical for the ultimate success of dental implants. I accept responsibility for any adverse consequences which result from not following my dentist's advice.

Questions I have to ask my dentist:

I HAVE READ AND FULLY UNDERSTAND THIS AUTHORIZATION AND CONSENT TO IMPLANT PLACEMENT AND ANESTHESIA, AND ALL MY QUESTIONS IF ANY, HAVE BEEN FULLY ANSWERED. I HAVE HAD THE OPPORTUNITY TO TAKE THIS DOCUMENT HOME AND REVIEW IT BEFORE SIGNING. I UNDERSTAND AND AGREE THAT MY INITIAL ON EACH PAGE, ALONG WITH MY SIGNATURE BELOW, ESTABLISHES THAT I HAVE GIVEN MY INFORMED CONSENT TO PROCEED WITH TREATMENT.

Dentist Signature (Print Name) _____

Witness Signature (Print Name) _____

Patient Signature (Print Name) _____

Parent or Guardian, if Patient is a Minor

2 Maxillary Sinus Augmentation Consent

Consent for Sinus Augmentation Procedure

Diagnosis. After a careful oral examination and study of my dental condition, my periodontist has advised me that my missing tooth or teeth may be replaced with artificial teeth supported by an implant.

Recommended Treatment. In order to treat my condition, my dentist has recommended the use of root form dental implants. I understand that the procedure for root form implants involves placing implants into the jawbone. As extraction of teeth underneath my sinuses will result in bone erosion or loss, a necessary procedure will be required for increasing the bone height in order to successfully place the implants. This procedure is called maxillary sinus augmentation.

Surgical Phase of Procedure. I understand that sedation may be utilized and that a local anesthetic will be administered to me as part of the treatment.

My gum tissue will be opened to expose the bone covering the maxillary sinus or sinuses. This bone has to be drilled to get access to the maxillary sinus. The internal tissue lining of the sinus will be elevated into a higher position and kept in there by adding bone. The source of bone will vary and may be from human, animal, or artificial sources.

Depending upon the case, implants will be placed at the same time by drilling through my jawbone and partially embedding into the bone graft of the maxillary sinus.

The gum and soft tissue will be stitched, closed over or around the implants. A periodontal bandage or dressing may be placed. Healing will be allowed to proceed for a period of 6 to 12 months. I understand that dentures usually cannot be worn during the first 1 to 2 weeks of the healing phase.

I further understand that if clinical conditions turn out to be unfavorable for the use of the sinus augmentation or prevent the placement of implants, my dentist will make a professional judgment on the management of the situation. The procedure also may involve supplemental bone grafts or other types of grafts to build up the ridge of my jaw and thereby to assist in placement, closure, and security of my implant.

Expected Benefits. The purpose of sinus augmentation is to allow me to have more bone in order to place the implants.

Principal Risks and Complications. I understand that some patients do not respond successfully to the sinus augmentation procedure, and in such cases, the bone may be lost or implant surgery may not be successful in providing artificial teeth. Because each patient's condition is unique, long-term success may not occur.

I understand that complications may result from the bone augmentation or implant surgery, drugs, and anesthetics.

These complications include, but are not limited to: postsurgical infection; bleeding; swelling and pain; facial discoloration; transient but on occasion permanent numbness of the lip, tongue, teeth, chin, or gum; jaw joint injuries or associated muscle spasm; transient but on occasion permanent increased tooth looseness; tooth sensitivity to hot, cold, sweet, or acidic foods; shrinkage of the gum upon healing, resulting in elongation of some teeth and greater spaces between some teeth; cracking or bruising of the corners of the mouth; restricted ability to open my mouth for several days or weeks; impact on well-being; allergic reactions; injury to teeth; bone fractures; nasal sinus penetrations; delayed healing; and accidental swallowing of foreign matter. The exact duration of any complications cannot be determined, and they may be irreversible.

Patient Consent

I have been fully informed of the nature of sinus augmentation surgery, the procedure to be utilized, the risks and benefits of the surgery, the alternative treatments available, and the necessity for follow-up and self-care. I have had an opportunity to ask any questions I may have in connection with the treatment and to discuss my concerns with my dentist. After thorough deliberation, I hereby consent to the performance of sinus augmentation surgery as presented to me during consultation and in the treatment plan presentation as described in this document.

I also consent to use of another method if clinical conditions are found to be unfavorable. If clinical conditions prevent the use of the sinus augmentation procedure, I defer to my dentist's judgment on the surgical management of that situation. I also give my permission to receive supplemental bone grafts to build up the ridge of my jaw and thereby to assist in placement, closure, and security of my implants.

I CERTIFY THAT I HAVE READ AND
FULLY UNDERSTAND THIS DOCUMENT.

Date   (Printed Name of Patient, Parent, or Guardian)

Date   (Printed Name of Witness)

Consent for Oral Conscious Sedation

Diagnosis: I have been informed that my treatment can be performed with a variety of types of anesthesia. These include local anesthesia as normally used for minor dental treatment, local anesthesia supplemented with conscious oral sedation, and general anesthesia in the hospital or outpatient surgical center. My dentist has recommended oral sedation, in addition to other possible forms of anesthetic, because a long and stressful procedure is to be undertaken, certain medical or physical conditions of mine may so indicate, or I am subject to significant anxiety and emotional stress related to dental procedures.

Recommended Treatment: I understand that in oral conscious sedation, small doses of various medications will be taken intraorally by me to produce a state of relaxation, reduced perception of pain, and drowsiness; however, I will not be put to sleep as with a general anesthetic. In addition, local anesthetics will be administered to numb the areas of my mouth to be operated and thus further control pain. I understand that the drugs to be used may include:_____

I recognize that I must do several things in connection with oral sedation. Specifically, I must not drink any alcoholic beverage or take certain medications for 12 hours before and 24 hours after the procedure. Furthermore, I will arrange for a responsible adult to drive me home and stay with me until the effects of sedation have worn off. I will not drive a motor vehicle or operate dangerous machinery on the day that I will receive the sedation.

Expected Benefits: The purpose of the oral sedation is to lessen the significant and undesirable side effects of long stressful procedures by chemically reducing the fear and apprehension associated with these procedures.

Principal Risks and Complications: I understand that occasionally complications may be associated with oral conscious sedation. These include pain, nausea, vomiting, and allergic reaction. To help minimize risks and complications, I have disclosed to my dentist any drugs and medications that I am taking. I have also disclosed any abnormalities in my current physical status or past medical history. This include any history of drug or alcohol abuse and any reactions to medications or anesthetics.

Alternatives to Suggested Treatment: Alternatives to oral conscious sedation include a local anesthesia, IV sedation, intramuscular sedation, and general anesthesia in the hospital or a surgery center, either as an inpatient or as an outpatient. Local anesthesia and oral sedation may, however, not adequately dispel my fear, anxiety, or stress. If certain medical conditions are present, it may present greater risks. There may be less control of proper dosage with oral sedation than with IV sedation. General anesthesia will cause me to lose consciousness and generally involves greater risks than IV sedation.

Necessary Follow-up Care and Self-Care: I understand that I must refrain from drinking alcoholic beverages and taking certain medications for a 24-hour period following the administration of oral conscious sedation. I understand that responsible adults should drive me home and remain with me until the effects of the sedation have worn off, and that I should not drive or operate dangerous machinery for the remainder of the day on which I receive sedation.

No Warranty or Guarantee: I hereby acknowledge that no guarantee, warranty, or assurance has been given to me that the proposed treatment will be successful. I recognize that, as noted above, there are risks and potential complications in the administration of oral conscious sedation.

Publication of Records: I authorize photos, slides, or any viewing of my care and treatment during or after its completion to be used for the advancement of dentistry and reimbursement purposes. My identity will not be revealed to the general public, however, without my permission.

Patient Consent

I have been fully informed of the nature of oral conscious sedation, the risks and the benefits of this form of sedation, the alternatives available, and the necessity for follow-up. I have had the opportunity to ask any questions I may have in connection with the procedure and to discuss my concerns with my dentist. After thorough deliberation, I hereby consent to the use of oral conscious sedation as presented to me during consultation and in the treatment plan presentation as described in this document.

I CERTIFY THAT I HAVE READ AND FULLY UNDERSTAND THIS DOCUMENT.

Date   (Printed Name of Patient, Parent, or Guardian)

Date   (Printed Name of Witness)

4   Dental Extraction Consent

Consent for Extraction of Teeth

I hereby authorize my dentist to treat the *condition(s)* described below.

The procedure(s) planned to treat the condition(s) have been explained to me, and I understand the procedure(s) to be:

Extraction of teeth is an irreversible process and, whether routine or difficult, is a surgical procedure. As in any surgery, there are some risks. They include, but are not limited to, the following:

1. Swelling, bruising, and/or discomfort in the surgery and surrounding area
2. Stretching of the corners of the mouth resulting in cracking or bruising
3. Possible infection and/or delayed healing requiring additional treatment
4. Dry socket or severe jaw pain beginning a few days after surgery, usually requiring additional care
5. Possible damage to adjacent teeth, especially those with large fillings, caps, or crowns
6. Numbness or altered sensations in the teeth, gums, lip, tongue, and chin, due to the closeness of tooth roots (especially wisdom teeth) to the nerves,

which can be bruised or damaged. Almost always, sensation returns to normal, but in rare cases the loss may be permanent.

7. Limited jaw opening due to inflammation, muscle soreness, and/or swelling most commonly occurs after wisdom tooth removal. Sometimes it is related to stress on the jaw joints (TMJ), especially when TMJ problems already exist. Uncommonly, TMJ injury could occur.

8. Bleeding: Prolonged or heavy bleeding that may require additional treatment

9. Sharp ridges or bone splinters may form later at the edge of the socket. These usually require another surgery to smooth or remove.

10. Incomplete removal of tooth fragments to avoid injury to vital structures such as nerves or sinus; sometimes small root tips may be left in place.

11. Sinus injury: The roots of upper back teeth are often close to the sinus, and sometimes a piece of root can be displaced into the sinus or an opening may occur from the mouth into the sinus, which may require additional care, including surgery. The sinus could become infected and require medical treatment and/or sinus surgery.

12. Periodontal (supporting bone and gum) defect that compromises health of adjacent tooth.

13. Jaw fracture: While quite rare, it is possible in a difficult extraction, especially of deeply impacted teeth.

14. Allergic reactions (previously unknown) to any medications used in treatment.

15. The risks of local anesthetic (numbing medicine) include soreness, bruising, infection, and allergic reactions.

16. Medications, drugs, anesthetics, and prescriptions may cause drowsiness and lack of awareness and coordination, which could be increased by the use of alcohol or other drugs. You should be with a responsible caretaker and should not drive, operate complicated machinery or devices, or make important decisions such as signing documents.

17. Smoking cigarettes increases the chances of delayed healing, dry socket, and periodontal, sinus, and anesthetic complications.

My dentist and I have discussed the nature of the problem(s) being treated, the planned procedure(s), alternative treatment options, and the risks associated with the treatment and alternative options. I understand that no guarantee can be promised, and I give my free and voluntary consent for treatment. I realize that my doctor may discover conditions requiring different surgery from that which was planned, and I give my permission for those additional procedures that are advisable in the exercise of professional judgment.

I understand that following extractions, teeth may shift and alter my bite. Loss of teeth could also affect my nutritional and general health, unless such teeth were in positions that were not useful. Consultation with my general dentist for prosthetic replacement is advised.

My signature below signifies that all questions have been answered to my satisfaction regarding this consent, and I fully understand the risks involved of the proposed surgery and anesthesia. I have given a complete and truthful medical history, including all medications, drug use, allergies, pregnancy, etc.

Patient's (or Legal Guardian's) Signature   Date

Doctor's Signature   Date

Witness' Signature   Date

5   Ridge Augmentation Consent

Consent for Ridge Augmentation Bone Graft Procedure

Diagnosis. After a careful oral examination and study of my dental condition my dentist, has advised me that my missing tooth or teeth may be replaced with artificial teeth supported by an implant,

Recommended Treatment. In order to treat my condition my dentist, has recommended the use of root form dental implants. I understand that the procedure for root form implants involves placing implants into the jawbone. As extraction of teeth will result in bone erosion or loss, a necessary procedure will be required for increasing the bone height or width in order to successfully place the implants. This procedure is called ridge augmentation bone graft.

Surgical Phase of Procedure. I understand that sedation may be utilized and that a local anesthetic will be administered to me as part of the treatment.

My gum tissue will be opened to expose the bone where implants to be placed. Then bone graft material will be added to the deficient area of my jawbone. The source of that bone will be human, animal or artificial. It is also possible that the bone will be harvested from other areas of my mouth.

Depending upon the case implants may be placed at the same time by drilling through my jawbone and partially embedding into the bone graft.

The gum and soft tissue will be stitched closed over or around the implants. A periodontal bandage or dressing may be placed. Healing will be allowed to proceed for a period of three to six months. I understand that dentures usually cannot be worn during the first one to two weeks of the healing phase.

I further understand that if clinical conditions turn out to be unfavorable for the use of the bone graft or prevent the placement of implants. My dentist, will make a professional judgment on the management of the situation. The procedure also may involve supplemental bone grafts or other types of grafts to build up the ridge of my jaw and thereby to assist in placement, closure, and security of my implants,

Expected Benefits. The purpose of ridge augmentation *graft* procedure is to allow me to have more bone in order to place the implants.

Principal Risks and Complications. I understand that some patients do not respond successfully to the bone graft procedure, and in such cases, the bone may be lost or implant surgery may not be successful in providing artificial teeth. Because each patient's condition is unique, long-term success may not occur.

I understand that complications may result from the bone augmentation or implant surgery, drugs, and anesthetics

These complications include, but are not limited to, post-surgical infection, bleeding, swelling and pain, facial discoloration, transient but on occasion permanent numbness of the lip, tongue, teeth, chin or gum, jaw joint injuries or associated muscle spasm, transient but on occasion permanent increased tooth looseness, tooth sensitivity to hot, cold, sweet or acidic foods, shrinkage of the gum upon healing resulting in elongation of some teeth and greater spaces between some teeth, cracking or bruising of the comers of the mouth, restricted ability to open the mouth for several days or weeks, impact on speech, allergic reactions, injury to teeth, bone fractures, nasal and maxillary sinus penetrations, maxillary sinus infection and bleeding, delayed healing, and accidental swallowing of foreign matter. The exact duration of any complications cannot be determined, and they may be irreversible.

Alternatives to Suggested Treatment. Alternative treatments for missing teeth include no treatment 'new removable appliances, and other procedures depending on the circumstances. However, continued. Wearing of ill-fitting and loose removable appliances can result in further damage to the bone and soft tissue of my mouth.

Necessary Follow-up Care. I understand that it is important for me to continue to see my dentist or prosthodontist. Implants, natural teeth and appliances have to be maintained daily in a clean, hygienic manner. Implants and appliances must also be examined periodically and may need to be adjusted. I understand that it is important for me to abide by the specific prescriptions and instructions given by my dentist

No Warranty or Guarantee. I hereby acknowledge that no guarantee, warranty or assurance has been given to me that the proposed treatment will be successful. Due to individual patient differences, a dentist cannot predict certainty of success. There exists the risk of failure, relapse, additional treatment, or worsening of my present condition, including the possible loss of certain teeth, despite the best of care.

Publication of Records. I authorize photos, slides, X-rays or any other viewing of my care and treatment during or after its completion to be used for the advancement of dentistry and for reimbursement purposes. My identity will not be revealed to the general public, however, without my permission.

Patient Consent

I have been fully informed of the *nature* of ridge augmentation bone graft surgery, the procedure to be utilized, the risks and benefits of the surgery, the alternative treatments available, and the necessity for follow-up and self-care. I have had an opportunity to ask any questions I may have in connection with the treatment and to discuss my concerns with my dentist. After thorough deliberation, I hereby consent to the performance of ridge augmentation bone graft surgery as presented to me during consultation and in the treatment plan presentation as described in this document.

I also consent to use of another method if clinical conditions are found to be unfavorable. If clinical conditions prevent the use of the bone graft procedure, I defer to my dentist's judgment on the surgical management of that situation. I also give my permission to receive supplemental bone grafts to build up the ridge of my jaw and thereby to assist in placement, closure, and security of my implants.

I CERTIFY THAT I HAVE READ AND
FULLY UNDERSTAND THIS DOCUMENT.

Date   (Printed Name of Patient, Parent, or Guardian)

Date   (Printed Name of Witness)

6   Bisphosphonates Consent

Consent for Oral Surgical Treatment in Patients Who Have Received Oral Bisphosphonate Drugs

Patient's Name   Date

Please initial each paragraph after reading. If you have any questions, please ask your doctor BEFORE initialing.

Having been treated previously with oral bisphosphonate drugs, you should know that there is a very small, but real, risk of future complications associated with dental treatment. This risk is currently estimated to be less than 1/10 of one percent. Bisphosphonate drugs appear to adversely affect the health of jaw bones, thereby reducing or eliminating the jaw bones' ordinarily excellent healing capacity. This risk is increased after surgery, especially from extraction, implant placement, or other "invasive" procedures that might cause even mild trauma to the bone. Spontaneous exposure of the jaw bone (osteonecrosis) may result. This is a smoldering, long-term, destructive process in the jawbone that is often very difficult or impossible to eliminate.

Your medical/dental history is _very_ important. We must know the medications and drugs that you have received or taken or are currently receiving or taking. An accurate medical history, including names of physicians, is important.

The decision to discontinue oral bisphosphonate drug therapy before dental treatment should be made by you in consultation with your medical doctor.

1. If a complication occurs, antibiotic therapy may be used to help control infection. For some patients, such therapy may cause allergic responses or have undesirable side effects such as gastric discomfort, diarrhea, colitis, etc.

2. Despite all precautions, there may be delayed healing, osteonecrosis, loss of bone and soft tissues, pathologic fracture of the jaw, an oral-cutaneous fistula (open draining wound), or other significant complications.

3. If osteonecrosis should occur, treatment may be prolonged and difficult, involving ongoing intensive therapy, including hospitalization, long-term antibiotics, and debridement to remove non-vital bone. Reconstructive surgery may be required, including bone grafting, metal plates and screws, and/or skin flaps and grafts.

4. Even if there are no immediate complications from the proposed dental treatment, the area is always subject to spontaneous breakdown and infection due to the condition of the bone. Even minimal trauma from a toothbrush, chewing hard food, or denture sores may trigger a complication.

5. Long-term postoperative monitoring may be required, and cooperation in keeping scheduled appointments is important. Regular and frequent dental check-ups with your dentist are important to monitor and attempt to prevent breakdown in your oral health.

6. I have read the above paragraphs and understand the possible risks of undergoing my planned treatment. I understand and agree to the following treatment plan.

7. I understand the importance of my health history and affirm that I have given any and all information that may impact my care. I understand that failure to give true health information may adversely affect my care and lead to unwanted complications.

8. I realize that, despite all precautions that may be taken to avoid complications, there can be no guarantee as to the result of the proposed treatment.

Consent

I certify that I speak, read, and write English and have read and fully understand this consent for surgery; that I have had my questions answered; and that all blanks were filled in prior to my initials or signature.

Patient's (or Legal Guardian's) Signature   Date

Doctor's Signature   Date

Witness' Signature   Date

7 Biopsy Consent

Informed Consent for Biopsy with Local Anesthesia

I understand that due to the type of lesion I have, my dentist has recommended that I undergo a biopsy, which is a procedure in which a portion of the lesion will be removed. The expected result of this procedure is to adequately diagnose the lesion type.

I understand that there are risks and complications associated with this procedure, which include but are not limited to infection, the need for another biopsy to be performed, and scarring.

Understanding all of the above, I request that and hereby provide my informed consent to the treating doctor and his/her assistants to perform a biopsy. I understand that, in the course of the biopsy, it may become necessary to perform additional procedures which are not known to be needed at this time. I request that and hereby provide my informed consent to the treating doctor to perform such procedures at his/her discretion if needed during my biopsy.

I consent to having local anesthesia. I understand the performance of diagnostic studies relating to my biopsy will be performed by other medical/dental professionals.

I confirm with my signature that:

- My dentist has discussed the above information with me.
- I have had the chance to ask questions.
- All of my questions have been answered to my satisfaction.
- I do hereby consent to the treatment described in this form.

Signature of Responsible Party   Date

Relationship to Party (if Responsible Party is Not Patient)

I confirm with my signature that I have discussed with the above-named patient the risks, potential complications, and intended benefits of the biopsy, as well as alternatives. The patient has had the opportunity to ask questions, all questions have been answered, and the patient has expressed understanding. Thus informed, the patient has requested that I perform a biopsy upon him/her.

Signature of Dentist   Date

Witness to Signatures Only   Date

8   Blank Consent Form

[r]Permission for Dental Procedure(s)

I hereby authorize my dentist to perform upon me or the named patient the following procedure(s): _____

My dentist has fully explained to me the purpose of the procedure(s) and has also informed me of expected benefits complications (from known to unknown cause), attendant discomforts and risks that may rise, as well as possible alternatives to the proposed treatment, including not treatment. The attendant risks of no treatment have been discussed. I have given an opportunity to ask questions, and all my questions have been answered fully and satisfactorily.

I understand that during the course of the procedure(s), unforeseen condition may arise which necessitate procedure(s) that my dentist may consider necessary.

I acknowledge that no guarantees or assurances have been made to me concerning the results intended from the procedure(s).

I confirm that I have read fully and understand the above and that all blank spaces have been completed prior to signing.

Patient/Relative or Guardian:

Signature   Print Name   Date
Relationship (if signed by person other than patient

Witness Signature   Print Name   Date

Dentist Certification:

I hereby certify that I explain the nature, purpose, benefits, risks of and alternatives to (including no treatment and attendant), the proposed procedure(s). I have offered to answer any questions and have fully answered all such questions. I believed that the patient/relative/guardian fully understands what I have explained and answered.

Dentist's Signature   Printed Name   Date

9   Gingivectomy Consent

Patient Consent form Gingivectomy

We would like our patients to be informed about the various procedures involved in periodontal therapy before you consent to treatment.

Facts about Gum Growths: Gum tissue will grow in response to hormonal changes, infection, medications, plaque, tumors, and trauma. As the gums grow it may make it difficult to clean your teeth properly. Bacterial plaque on tooth surfaces under the gum causes a loss of bone supporting the tooth.

Treatment Plan alternatives: Surgically reducing this extra tissue allows for access for oral hygiene and reduces the risk for infection.

Risks: Complications of treatment include (but are not limited to): bleeding or infection which is temporary, but on rare occasions may require further treatment. Therapy may result in gum recession, exposure of metal crown margins, sensitivity to hot or cold temperatures, and on rare occasions may cause numbness or tingling sensations in and around the mouth, TMJ (jaw joint disorders), or the loss of teeth.

No treatment Risk: Pain or infection which may result in a loss of teeth and would require further treatment.

All questions about the proposed treatment, alternatives to the proposed treatment, and the risks involved have been answered to my satisfaction. I authorize my dentist and his staff to perform the treatment and any emergency treatment that my dentist believes to be appropriate. I understand that the proposed treatment contains no guarantee of success. I understand that I may refuse to consent to any and all treatment.

Signature Patient/Guardian _____

Date

Witness

_____

Date

10   Gingival Augmentation Consent

Consent for Gingival Augmentation Surgery

Diagnosis. After a careful oral examination and study of my dental condition my dentist, has advised me that I have significant gum recession. I understand that with this condition, further recession of the gum may occur. In addition, for fillings at the gum line or crowns with edges under the gum line, it is important to have sufficient width of attached gum to withstand the irritation caused by the fillings or edges of crowns. Gum tissue may also be placed to improve appearance and to protect roots of the teeth.

Recommended Treatment. In order to treat this condition my dentist, has recommended that gingival augmentation procedures be performed in areas of my mouth with significant gum recession. I understand that sedation may be utilized and that a local anesthetic will be administered to me as part of the treatment. This surgical procedure involves the transplanting of a thin strip of gum from the roof of my mouth, from the adjacent teeth or from a tissue bank (Allograft). The transplanted strip of gum can be placed at the base of the remaining gum, or it can be placed so as to partially cover the tooth root surface exposed by the recession. A periodontal bandage or dressing may be placed.

Expected Benefits. The purpose of gingival augmentation is to create an amount of attached gum tissue adequate to reduce the likelihood of further gum recession. Another purpose for this procedure may be to cover exposed root surfaces, to enhance the appearance of the teeth and gum line, or to prevent or treat root sensitivity or root decay.

Principal Risks and Complications. I understand that a small number of patients do not respond successfully to gingival augmentation. If a transplant is placed so as to partially cover the tooth root surface exposed by the recession, the gum placed over the root may shrink back during healing. In such a case, the attempt to cover the exposed root surface may not be completely successful. Indeed, in some cases, it may result in more recession with increased spacing between the teeth.

I understand that complications may result from gingival augmentation or from anesthetics. These complications include, but are not limited to: (1) postsurgical infection; (2) bleeding, swelling, and pain; (3) facial discoloration; (4) transient, or on occasion permanent, tooth sensitivity to hot, cold, sweet, or acidic foods; (5) allergic reactions; and (6) accidental swallowing of foreign matter. The exact duration of any complications cannot be determined, and they may be irreversible.

There is no method that will accurately predict or evaluate how my gum and bone will heal. I understand that there may be a need for a second procedure if the initial surgery is not satisfactory. In addition, the success of gingival augmentation can be affected by (1) medical conditions, (2) dietary and nutritional problems, (3) smoking, (4) alcohol consumption, (5) clenching and grinding of teeth, (6) inadequate oral hygiene, and (7) medications that I may be taking. To my knowledge, I have reported to the dentist any prior drug reactions, allergies, diseases, symptoms, habits, or conditions which might in any way relate to this surgical procedure. I understand that my diligence in providing the personal daily care recommended by my dentist, and taking all prescribed medications, are important to the ultimate success of the procedure.

Alternatives to Suggested Treatment. My dentist has explained alternative treatments for my gum recession. These include no treatment, continued monitoring for progressive recession, and modification of technique for brushing my teeth.

Necessary Follow-up Care and Self-Care. I understand that it is important for me to continue to see my regular dentist. Existing restorative dentistry can be an important factor in the success or failure of gingival augmentation.

I recognize that natural teeth and appliances should be maintained daily in a clean, hygienic manner. I will need to come for appointments following my surgery so that my healing may be monitored and so that my dentist can evaluate and report on the outcome of surgery upon completion of healing. Smoking or alcohol intake may adversely affect gum healing and may limit the successful outcome of my surgery. I know that it is important (1) to abide by the specific prescriptions and instructions given by the dentist, and (2) to see my dentist for periodic examination and preventive treatment. Maintenance also may include adjustment of prosthetic appliances.

No Warranty or Guarantee. I hereby acknowledge that no guarantee, warranty, or assurance has been given to me that the proposed treatment will be successful. In most cases, the treatment should provide benefit in reducing the cause of my condition and should produce healing which will help me keep my teeth. Due to individual patient differences, however, a dentist cannot predict certainty of success. There is risk of failure, relapse, additional treatment, or even worsening of my present condition, including the possible loss of certain teeth, despite the best of care.

Publication of Records. I authorize photos, slides, x-rays, or any other viewings of my care and treatment during or after its completion to be used for the advancement of dentistry and reimbursement purposes. My identity will not be revealed to the general public, however, without my permission.

Patient Consent

I have been fully informed of the nature of gingival augmentation surgery, the procedure to be utilized, the risks and benefits of periodontal surgery, the alternative treatments available, and the necessity for follow-up and self-care. I have had an opportunity to ask any questions I may have in connection with the treatment and to discuss my concerns with the dentist. After thorough deliberation, I hereby consent to the performance of gingival augmentation surgery as presented to me during consultation, and in the treatment plan presentation as described in this document. I also consent to the performance of such additional or alternative procedures as may be deemed necessary in the best judgment of my dentist

I CERTIFY THAT I HAVE READ AND
FULLY UNDERSTAND THIS DOCUMENT.

Date   (Printed Name of Patient, Parent, or Guardian)

Date   (Printed Name of Witness)

Part B: Sample Surgical Report

OPERATIVE REPORT

DATE:
PATIENT:

Preoperative Diagnosis: Pneumatized bilateral maxillary sinuses and posterior missing teeth.

Postoperative Diagnosis: Augmentation of the bilateral maxillary sinuses and three endosseous implants.

Assistant:
Surgeon:

PROCEDURE: Bilateral maxillary sinus augmentation together with insertion of implants #3, 12, and 13.

PROCEDURE IN DETAIL: The patient was brought to the operatory around 11:00 am. She was premedicated with Halcion 0.125 mg one tablet one hour prior to the procedure. She was placed in a chair in the semi-supine position. Next, four carpules of xylocaine 1:100,000 epinephrine, approximately 4 cc, were injected to the buccal and lingual of the maxillary bilateral posterior area for the purpose of hemostasis and analgesia. This was followed by a crestal incision in the #3 and 4 areas together with a vertical buccal releasing incision with reflection of a full-thickness mucoperiosteal flap. This was followed by designing of the window osteotomy to be approximately 6 mm wide × 5 mm high, and reflected with no complications and no perforation of the Schneiderian membrane. At this time, the initial osteotomy was started using the surgical stent until the final diameter and length were reached. This was followed by insertion of a Straumann SLA bone level (4.8 mm in diameter, 10 mm in length) with no complications. The tip of the implant was augmented into the window osteotomy using Puros Putty freeze-demineralized bone allograft with bone chips approximately 0.25 cc, followed by covering the window with DynaMatrix collagen membrane. Suturing was accomplished using a PTFE 4-0 continuous sling and covered with surgical glue. At this time, attention was turned to the #12 and 13 areas, where the exact procedure was rendered crestal incision in the #12 and 13 areas with buccal vertical releasing incision #12 buccal with a different size window which was approximately 8 mm in width × 6 mm in height and again no visible perforation of the Schneiderian membrane. Implants 12 and 13 were placed, which were Straumann bone level SLA (4.8 mm in diameter, 10 mm in length) for both of them, and the bone used for augmenting around the implant tips and the window was Puros Putty freeze-demineralized bone allograft with bone chips approximately 0.5 cc. Suturing was accomplished using a PTFE 4-0 continuous sling and covered with surgical glue. Periapical films were taken that showed good position of the implants in relationship to the neighboring teeth, and the bone mass around the implants into the augmented sinus. Postoperative instructions were given in addition to ice pack.

Prescriptions: Levaquin 500 mg one tab q.d. #10 tablets, Oxycodone 5 mg one tab q 6h p.r.n. pain #10 tablets, Motrin 800 mg one tab q 6h p.r.n. pain #20 tablets, and Medrol Dosepak to use as directed, no refills. The patient was advised to monitor her blood sugar level while taking the Medrol Dosepack.

Postoperative instructions were given in addition to the sinus augmentation instructions and discussed with the patient's granddaughter.

This marked the end of the surgical procedure. The patient tolerated the procedure very well. She was dismissed alert and showed no sign of distress upon dismissal.

Signed by Surgeon:

Part C: Sample Postoperative Instructions and How to Clean Implants

POSTOPERATIVE INSTRUCTIONS

DISCOMFORT AND MEDICATIONS: Periodontal surgery, like other surgical procedures, may be associated with varying degrees of discomfort. This depends on the procedure involved and individual differences. If analgesics have been pre-scribed, it is usual to take the first dose while the surgical site is still anesthetized ("numb"). All medication should be taken strictly as prescribed. The interval between taking the medications and the total length of time that you are to remain on your medications have been carefully determined to give you the maximum benefit with the minimum use of drugs. Variation from the prescribed regime can affect healing and the success of your procedure.

BLEEDING: You may notice slight bleeding from the surgical site. This type of minor bleeding for one or two days is not unusual and is not a major concern. If at any time you notice the formation of large blood clots or any obvious flow of blood which is more than light ooze, notify your doctor at once.

SUTURES: Sutures ("stitches") are placed to hold the gingival tissues in the proper position for ideal healing. If sutures ("stitches") were placed, your doctor will usually want you to return so that they can be fully removed once sufficient healing has occurred. Do not disturb the sutures with your tongue or toothbrush, or in any other manner, since displacement will impair healing. If you notice that a suture has come out or come loose, notify your doctor during regular office hours.

DRESSING: A periodontal dressing is often used to cover the surgical site for one to two weeks after surgery. The dressing is placed around your teeth to protect the surgical area and should not be disturbed. If small pieces become lost, and you have no discomfort, there is no cause for concern. If large pieces break off or the entire dressing becomes loose in the first 2–4 days, please contact the dentist.

DIET: For your comfort and to protect the surgical area, a soft diet is recom-mended. Avoid chewing in the area of surgery. Avoid hard, fibrous, or "sharp" foods (such as corn chips) as these may be uncomfortable and can dislodge the periodontal dressing. Drink plenty of liquids. It is important to maintain a diet with a normal calorie level that is high in protein, minerals, and vitamins to sup-port postoperative healing. Eat as normal a diet as possible. POSTSURGICALLY IS NOT THE TIME TO START A DIET, since this can have detrimental effects on healing and lessen the chances of success of the surgical therapy.

ORAL HYGIENE: Continue to brush and floss the teeth that were not involved in the surgery (or covered by the periodontal dressing). The surgical area should not be disturbed for the first week postoperatively. However, you may rinse gen-tly with salt water or with a mouthwash if prescribed by your doctor. After your sutures have been removed, generally after 1 week, you should lightly clean the teeth using a soft toothbrush or as instructed by your doctor. The gentle applica-tion of a fluoride gel with your toothbrush will also help to control plaque.

PHYSICAL ACTIVITY: Avoid strenuous physical activity during your immedi-ate recovery period, usually 2 to 3 days.

SWELLING: Some slight swelling of the operated area is not unusual and may begin after the surgery. An ice pack may be used to minimize swelling. Ice should be placed in a plastic bag, and then wrapped in a thick cloth towel and applied directly over the surgical area. You should maintain the towel-wrapped ice pack in contact with the skin as much as possible for the first 24 hours after surgery. You should also keep your head elevated above the level of your heart during the first

24 hours after surgery. This may necessitate the use of several pillows to support your head and upper body while sleeping. If swelling occurs, it usually disappears after several days. Applying moist heat to the swollen area will help the swelling resolve; however, heat should not be applied until at least 1–2 days after surgery. Any unusual or large swelling should be reported to your dentist at once.

SMOKING: All smoking should be stopped until after your sutures have been removed to ensure the best healing and success of your surgical procedure. Healing results are significantly worse in smokers than in nonsmokers.

ALCOHOL: All intake of alcohol should be stopped until after your sutures have been removed, and intake should be minimized for the next several weeks after suture removal to enhance healing. The combination of alcohol and certain pain medication is not recommended.

DO NOT'S: For the next several days, do NOT spit, smoke, rinse hard, drink through a straw, create a "sucking" action in your mouth, use a commercial mouth-wash, drink carbonated soda, or use an oral irrigating device.

HOW TO CLEAN IMPLANTS FORM

Having dental implants in your mouth requires more care and attention than natural teeth, which is due to the fact that the seal between the gum tissue and the implant surface is much weaker than that for your natural teeth. Research has shown that gingivitis around implants can destroy 70% of this seal. When this occurs, bacteria and bacterial products have a free path of entry to the bone which will eventually result in implant failure. It is very important to follow the regime described below to keep your implants clean and healthy.

Home Care Regime for Dental Implants

- Clean the implant at least twice a day, especially after breakfast and the last meal of the day. These times are especially important as saliva flow decreases during sleep, which allows bacterial accumulation.

Tooth-brushing options are:

a. Ultra-soft-bristle toothbrush
b. Motorized multitufted or unitufted toothbrush.

The following can provide effective yet gentle cleaning:

a. Low-abrasive commercial toothpaste
b. Floss, super floss, floss threader, pipe cleaners with synthetic bristles, or yarn (dip in Peridex)
c. Proxabrush with coated center wire and synthetic bristles
d. Disclosing tablets or solution to determine locations of plaque accumulation
e. Antimicrobial mouth rinses: Use Peridex or Listerine. Apply to implant neck with hand, motorized toothbrush, or floss dipped in it at least once daily. If you have tooth-colored fillings, avoid rinsing as it will discolor your fillings if used

for a long time. Be thorough but gentle. Clean the neck of the dental implant. Ask your hygienist to demonstrate the proper technique and angulation.

   f. Water Pic or other oral irrigation instrument: Because of its destructive potential, you should be carefully instructed in the use of oral irrigation. You should always select the lowest possible flow rate and never direct the stream at the gum of the implant junction.

This regime is specifically designed for implant patients. It is our belief that implant patients are the co-therapists in the implant procedure. The excellence required by the dentist demands that the patient be seen regularly to avoid potential problems that might lead to unexpected failure.

Part D: Sample Patient Letters

«Salutation»

We appreciate the trust you have placed in us by scheduling an appointment for a dental health evaluation. We are now making it possible for many of our patients to eat and speak with comfort and confidence through oral implants. Today, advanced diagnostic and treatment modalities are available.

Many patients have spaces where teeth were lost or removed. Traditional dental restorations aren't always the best solution for missing teeth. Implants prevent having to sacrifice the structure of surrounding good teeth to bridge a space. Implants are like teeth and provide a stable biting and chewing surface because your jawbone supports them. Add to this the fact that many patients suffer from health-related conditions, which may include distressing mouth sores, digestive problems from inadequate chewing, difficulty swallowing, and gagging. The first stage of digestion, chewing, is often impaired with serious consequences. Associated problems could be regarded as medically necessary and may be reimbursable under health or dental insurance. Contact your insurance carrier to discuss possible benefits.

One of our primary concerns will be to make you feel comfortable in our office. We welcome the opportunity to answer your questions or discuss any matters with you. Since some time has passed, we need you to call and update our office with your intentions. We need to keep accurate records and have not heard from you recently.

Please call our office to schedule an appointment. Our staff will assist you in every way. We look forward to seeing you very soon.

Respectfully,

«Salutation»

We were reviewing your file and noticed that you have not scheduled or kept a cleaning and exam appointment. I am concerned that you haven't scheduled an appointment since you have had your implants uncovered in this office.

I have designed this regimen specifically for implant patients. The patient must be examined regularly to avoid potential problems that might lead to an unexpected failure. I recommend recall cleaning appointment between your general dentist and our office every 3 months: two cleanings here and two cleanings there within 1 year. I must stress the need to take yearly x-rays to monitor the surrounding bone and tissue to maintain the oral health and add to the longevity of your dental implants. Dental implants, like natural teeth, can become periodontally diseased, and this is the reason I want your implants monitored so frequently.

Please take the time to call our office and make the necessary appointment today. We are looking forward to seeing you soon.

Respectfully,

Part E: Sample Letters to Physicians

Re: «Title»

Dear Doctor

«Title» «FName» «MI» «LName» presented to our office for dental care. A review of the medical history indicated that Aspirin 325 mg tabs is taken daily.

Proposed dental treatment, including periodontal and implant surgery, will result in bleeding. We have recommended discontinuation of the blood thinners 48 hours prior to treatment. Please advise us on this issue.

Your guidance in the medical management of this patient is appreciated.

Part F: Sample Letters to Referring Dentists

Dear Doctor,

Dental Implant Completion Report

We have completed the implant treatment on your patient.

Restorative objectives:
Crowns #18, 19

Restorative needs:
Same

Dental implants placed in the following area:

Position	Implant type	Diameter	Length	Prognosis
18, 19	Straumann Bone Level RC	4.8 mm	8 mm	V Good
Restorative comments:				
Patient has healing caps ready for the final impression				

Thank you for your referral and the confidence you have in us to treat your patients.

Sincerely,

Index